SELF-ASSESSMENT FOR
MRCP (PART 1)

Self-Assessment for MRCP (Part 1)

C. F. CORKE
MB, BS, MRCP, (UK), FFARCS,
FFICANZA, FANZCA
Director of Intensive Care,
The Geelong Hospital,
Geelong, Victoria, Australia

FOURTH EDITION

Blackwell
Science

© 1981, 1984, 1991, 1996 by
Blackwell Science Ltd
Editorial Offices:
Osney Mead, Oxford OX2 0EL
25 John Street, London WC1N 2BL
23 Ainslie Place, Edinburgh EH3 6AJ
238 Main Street, Cambridge
  Massachusetts 02142, USA
54 University Street, Carlton
  Victoria 3053, Australia

Other Editorial Offices:
Arnette Blackwell SA
  1, rue de Lille, 75007 Paris
  France

Blackwell Wissenschafts-Verlag GmbH
  Kurfürstendamm 57
  10707 Berlin, Germany

Feldgasse 13, A-1238 Wien
Austria

First published 1981
Second edition 1984
Third edition 1991
Fourth edition 1996

Set by Semantic Graphics, Singapore
Printed and bound in Great Britain
by Hartnolls Ltd, Bodmin, Cornwall

DISTRIBUTORS

  Marston Book Services Ltd
  PO Box 87
  Oxford OX2 0DT
  (*Orders*: Tel: 01865 791155
          Fax: 01865 791927
          Telex: 837515)

North America
  Blackwell Science, Inc.
  238 Main Street
  Cambridge, MA 02142
  (*Orders*: Tel: 800 215-1000
          617 876-7000
          Fax: 617 492-5263)

Australia
  Blackwell Science Pty Ltd
  54 University Street
  Carlton, Victoria 3053
  (*Orders*: Tel: 03 9347 0300
          Fax: 03 9349 3016)

A catalogue record for this title
is available from the British Library

ISBN 0-86542-937-5

Library of Congress
Cataloging-in-Publication Data

Corke, C. F.
    Self assessment for MRCP.
    Part 1/C.F. Corke. — 4th ed.
        p.   cm.
    Includes bibliographical references
    and index.
    ISBN 0-86542-937-5
    1. Medicine—Examinations,
    questions, etc.
    I. Title.
    RC58.C624   1996
    610'.76—dc20   95-32582
                                        CIP

Contents

Preface

New questions have been added, particularly covering areas of medicine which have assumed increased importance during the years since the last edition, and others have been omitted.

New questions include subjects such as pneumocystis, cyclosporin, prostaglandins and interleukins. Other questions have been altered and the Notes Sections changed and expanded as new information has emerged.

TO THE FIRST EDITION

There is no textbook for the MRCP (Part 1) examination. The smaller 'student' textbooks do not cover the necessary material in adequate depth and the larger textbooks are generally too long for the average candidate to hope to read.

This book contains multiple choice questions of a similar type to those encountered in the examination, but in addition, there is a Notes Section relating to each question. This represents a synopsis of the information to which the question refers.

The Notes may be used without reference to the questions as a source of information. Reading numerous multiple choice questions, especially in the period shortly before the examination, is likely to be detrimental (the untrue statements may be recalled incorrectly during the examination) and the Notes may be particularly useful during this period.

There is a reference in each case to an up-to-date, respected text where the candidate may validate the answer to the question or the information in the notes, or may further research the topic.

No book of this length can be comprehensive. However, the main topics have been covered and I hope that the concept of the synopsis (Notes) may be of help to candidates attempting to retain information derived from other sources.

There are no questions covering fields of statistics or psychiatry. The questions related to these subjects in the examination tend to be reasonably straightforward and the candidate who reads one of the shorter student textbooks on these subjects should be well-equipped to tackle these questions in the examination.

This book is in appreciation of the excellent assistance from Stephen Due and the library staff of the Geelong Hospital in respect of this and other projects.

References

Braunwald E (1992) *Heart Disease—A Textbook of Cardiovascular Medicine*, 4th edn. W.B. Saunders, Philadelphia.

Champion RH, Burton JL & Ebling FJG (1992) *Textbook of Dermatology*, 5th edn. Blackwell Scientific Publications, Oxford.

Crofton J & Douglas A (1989) *Respiratory Diseases*, 4th edn. Blackwell Scientific Publications, Oxford.

DeGroot LJ *et al.* (1995) *Endocrinology*, 3rd edn. W.B. Saunders, Philadelphia.

DeVita VT, Hellman S & Rosenberg SA (1993) *Cancer. Principles and Practice of Oncology*, 4th edn. Lippincott, Philadelphia.

Gilman AG, Rall TW, Niles AS & Taylor P (1990) *Goodman and Gilman's The Pharmacological Basis of Therapeutics*, 8th edn. Macmillan, New York.

Hart FD (ed.) (1985) *French' s Index of Differential Diagnosis*, 12th edn. John Wright, Bristol.

Kelley WN, Harris ED, Ruddy S & Sledge CB (1993) *Textbook of Rheumatology*, 4th edn. W.B. Saunders, Philadelphia.

Lachmann PJ, Peters DK, Rosen FS & Walport MJ (1993) *Clinical Aspects of Immunology*, 5th edn. Blackwell Scientific Publications, Oxford.

Lee GR, Bithell TC, Foerster J, Athens JW & Lukens JN (1993) *Wintrobe's Clinical Haematology*, 9th edn. Lea & Febiger, Philadelphia.

Maegraith BG (1989) *Adams and Maegraith Clinical Tropical Diseases*, 9th edn. Blackwell Scientific Publications, Oxford.

Mandell GL, Bennett JE & Dolin R (1995) *Principles and Practice of Infectious Diseases*, 4th edn. Churchill Livingstone, Edinburgh.

Schrier RW & Gottschalk CW (1993). *Diseases of the Kidney*, 5th edn. Little, Brown, Boston.

Scriver CR, Beaudet AL, Sly WS & Valle D (1989) *The Metabolic Basis of Inherited Disease*, 6th edn. McGraw-Hill, New York.

Sherlock S & Dooley J (1993) *Diseases of the Liver and Biliary System*, 9th edn. Blackwell Scientific Publications, Oxford.

Sleisenger MH & Fordtran JF (1993) *Gastrointestinal Disease. Patho-*

physiology, Diagnosis and Management, 5th edn. W.B. Saunders, Philadelphia.

Walton JN (1993) *Brain's Diseases of the Nervous System,* 10th edn. Oxford University Press, Oxford.

List of Abbreviations

2,3 DPG	2,3-diphosphoglycerate
AAC	antibiotic-associated colitis
ACE	angiotensin-converting enzyme
aCML	atypical chronic myeloid leukaemia
ACTH	adrenocorticotrophic hormone
ADH	antidiuretic hormone
ADPKD	autosomal dominant polycystic kidney disease
AIDS	acquired immunodeficiency syndrome
AIP	acute intermittent porphyria
ALA	aminolaevulinic acid
ALL	acute lymphoblastic leukaemia
AML	acute myeloid leukaemia
ANA	antinuclear antibody
ANCAs	antineutrophil cytoplasmic antibodies
ANF	antinuclear factor
ART	automated reagin test
AVP	arginine vasopressin
cAMP	cyclic adenosine monophosphate
C-ANCA	cytoplasmic ANCA
CCK	cholecystokinin
CK	creatine kinase
CLL	chronic lymphatic leukaemia
CML	chronic myeloid leukaemia
CMV	cytomegalovirus
CNS	central nervous system
CoA	coenzyme A
CPT-1	carnitine palmitoyltransferase I
CREST	calcinosis, Raynaud's, abnormal oesophageal motility, sclerodactyly, telangiectasia
CRH	corticotrophin releasing hormone
CRST	calcinosis, Raynaud's phenomena, sclerodactyly, telangectasia
CSF	cerebrospinal fluid

CT	computerized tomography
D_2	dopamine
DDAVP	*d*-desaminoarginine vasopressin
ECG	electrocardiogram
EHEC	enterohaemorrhagic *Escherichia coli*
EIEC	enteroinvasive *Escherichia coli*
EMG	electromyogram
EPEC	enteropathogenic *Escherichia coli*
ER	oestrogen receptor
ESR	erythrocyte sedimentation rate
ETEC	enterotoxigenic *Escherichia coli*
Fab	fragment antigen binding
Fc	fragment crystalline
FE_{Na}	fractional excretion of sodium
FEV_1	forced expiratory volume in 1 second
FLH	farmers' lung hay
FRC	functional residual capacity
FVC	forced vital capacity
FPC	familial colonic polyposis
GAD	glutamic acid decarboxylase
G6PD	glucose-6-phosphate dehydrogenase
GFR	glomerular filtration rate
GvHD	graft-versus-host disease
GN	glomerulonephritis
HbA_{1c}	glycosylated haemoglobin
HbF	fetal haemoglobin
HBV	hepatitis B virus
HCV	hepatitis C virus
HIV	human immunodeficiency virus
HLA	human leukocyte antigen
HOCM	hypertrophic obstructive cardiomyopathy
HSV1	herpes simplex virus type 1
IAA	insulin autoantibodies
ICA	islet cell antibodies
IDDM	insulin-dependent diabetes mellitus
IFN-α	α-interferon
IFN-β	β-interferon
IFN-γ	γ-interferon
IGF-I	insulin-like growth factor I
IgG	immunoglobulin G

IL-2	interleukin 2
IV	intravenous
LAMB	lentigines, atrial myxoma and blue naevi
LCAT	lecithin cholesterol acyl transferase
LDL	low-density lipoprotein
MAC	*Mycobacterium avium* complex
MCH	mean corpuscular haemoglobin
MCHC	mean corpuscular haemoglobin concentration
MCNS	minimal-change nephrotic syndrome
MCV	mean corpuscular volume
MEA	multiple endocrine adenomatosis
MEN	multiple endocrine neoplasia
MND	motor neuron disease
NAD	nicotinamide adenine dinucleotide
NADP	nicotinamide adenine dinucleotide phosphate
NAME	naevi, atrial myxoma, myxoid neurofibroma, ephelides
NF1	neurofibromatosis of the von Recklinghausen type
NK	natural killer
NSU	non-specific urethritis
OI	osteogenesis imperfecta
PAN	polyarteritis nodosa
P-ANCA	perinuclear ANCA
PBG	porphobilinogen
PCV	packed cell volume
PGF	prostaglandin F
PGI$_2$	prostacyclin
PGR	progesterone receptors
PHP	pseudohypoparathyroidism
PRA	plasma renin activity
PRV	polycythaemia rubra vera
PT	prothrombin time
PTH	parathyroid hormone
PTT	partial thromboplastin time
PUVA	psoralen, ultraviolet
RFI	renal failure index
RPR	rapid plasma reagin
rt-PA	recombinant tissue plasminogen activator
RV	residual volume
SBE	subacute infective endocarditis
SC	secretory component

SIADH	syndrome of inappropriate ADH secretion
SLE	systemic lupus erythematosus
TBG	thyroid-binding globulin
TIBC	total iron-binding capacity
TLC	total lung capacity
TPHA	*Treponema pallidum* haemagglutination
TmG	maximal capacity of renal tubules to reabsorb glucose
TPI	*Treponema pallidum* immobilization
TSAb	thyroid-stimulating antibody
TSH	thyroid-stimulating hormone
TSS	toxic shock syndrome
TSST	toxic shock syndrome toxin
UNa	urinary sodium
VC	vital capacity
VDRL	Venereal Disease Research Laboratory
VIP	vasoactive intestinal polypeptide
VMA	vanillylmandelic acid
VP	variegate porphyria
vWD	von Willebrand's disease
vWF	von Willebrand's factor

Part 1
Multiple Choice Questions

1. **Features of cystinuria include**
a. excessive urinary lysine excretion
b. accumulation of cystine in renal tubular cells
c. ectopia lentis (lens dislocation)
d. radiolucent urinary calculi
e. a useful therapeutic response to ammonium chloride administration

2. **Ketones**
a. can be utilized by skeletal muscle as an energy source
b. in the circulation in diabetic ketoacidosis are characterized by a high circulating level of acetoacetate with a relatively smaller quantity of β-hydroxybutyrate
c. produced in the liver during starvation are principally derived from long-chain fatty acids from triglyceride stores in adipose tissue
d. production is favoured by high glucagon levels
e. synthesis is inhibited by high intracellular concentrations of malonyl–coenzyme A (CoA)

3. **The corticospinal tract**
a. runs on the anterior aspect of the medulla
b. originates predominantly from the cortical cells of the precentral gyrus
c. does not run in the posterior limb of the internal capsule
d. runs in the pyramid
e. decussates in the midbrain

4. **Which of the following findings support a diagnosis of acute tubular necrosis rather than prerenal failure?**
a. urinary sodium concentration of 10 mmol/l
b. urine osmolality of 300 mosmol/kg
c. renal tubular epithelial cells on urine microscopy

d. renal failure index (RFI) of 1.5

e. the fractional excretion of sodium (FE_{Na}) of 10%

5. After infection with *Salmonella typhi*

a. children are especially likely to be carriers

b. most of those becoming carriers are male

c. faecal culture is almost always positive during the first week of illness

d. relapse does not occur if antibiotics (chloramphenicol) are taken for 2 weeks

e. the duration of enteric fever is not reduced by ampicillin treatment

6. Ptosis

a. results from damage to parasympathetic nerves which run with the oculomotor nerve

b. is associated with mydriasis when due to a complete third-nerve lesion

c. is associated with damage to the cervical sympathetic nervous system

d. is associated with paralysis of accommodation when due to damage to the oculomotor nerve

e. of congenital origin is almost invariably bilateral

7. In systemic lupus erythematosus (SLE)

a. antinuclear factor (ANF) is present in <75% of cases

b. lymphocytotoxic antibodies are rarely present in the serum of patients with untreated disease

c. antiphospholipid antibodies are associated with prolongation of the prothrombin time (PT)

d. decreased complement factor 2 is the most sensitive indicator of disease activity

e. increased suppressor T-cell function is a constant finding in active disease

8. Glycosylated haemoglobin

a. is pathognomonic of diabetes mellitus

b. is glycosylated haemoglobin A

c. formation is directly proportional to the time-average concentration of glucose within the erythrocyte

d. levels would be expected to fall within 2 weeks of excellent glucose control in a previously poorly-controlled diabetic

e. levels which are very high in early pregnancy are associated with increased risks of congenital abnormality in the babies

9. **Which of the following structures are situated in the midbrain?**
   a. the cerebral aqueduct
   b. the facial (VII) nucleus
   c. the nucleus ambiguus
   d. the red nucleus
   e. the superior colliculus

10. **Actions of cyclosporin include**
    a. depression of phagocytosis by hepatic macrophages
    b. increased interleukin 2 (IL-2) receptor expression by cytotoxic T cells
    c. enhanced proliferation of suppressor T cells
    d. enhanced IL-2 production by activated T cells
    e. enhanced helper T-cell response to IL-1

11. **In von Willebrand's disease**
    a. inheritance is predominantly autosomal recessive
    b. there is generally a deficiency of platelet adhesiveness
    c. thrombostasis is generally improved more by infusion of factor VIII concentrate than by cryoprecipitate
    d. *d*-desaminoarginine vasopressin (DDAVP) treatment causes a reduction of the bleeding time
    e. DDAVP therapy results in increased circulating levels of von Willebrand factor

12. **The oculomotor nerve**
    a. runs along the lateral wall of the cavernous sinus
    b. runs in close proximity to the posterior communicating artery
    c. innervates the lateral rectus muscle
    d. carries parasympathetic fibres
    e. runs over the apex of the petrous temporal bone

3

13. **A man known to have a carcinoma of the bronchus develops generalized pigmentation and muscle weakness, so**
    a. his carcinoma is probably of the 'oat-cell' type
    b. he probably has tumour replacement of his adrenals causing adrenal insufficiency
    c. a blood sugar value of 18 mmol/l would be inconsistent with the diagnosis
    d. hypokalaemia would be an expected finding
    e. he may be treated with aminoglutethimide

14. **Myasthenia gravis**
    a. is most likely to improve after thymectomy in those with a thymoma
    b. characteristically results in depression of tendon reflexes
    c. occurs most commonly in those over 50 years old
    d. circulating antiacetylcholine receptor antibody is found in <50% of adults with generalized active myasthenia gravis
    e. is associated with thyrotoxicosis

15. **Carbon dioxide retention**
    a. is associated with decreased cerebral blood flow
    b. results from pulmonary oedema
    c. is a cause of papilloedema
    d. is associated with hypotension
    e. is associated with coarse tremor

16. **Findings consistent with a diagnosis of untreated classic phenylketonuria include**
    a. microcephaly
    b. an IQ of 100
    c. a normal serum phenylalanine level at birth
    d. a marked elevation of blood tyrosine level after a phenylalanine challenge
    c. a low serum glycine level

17. **Which of the following statements are true with respect to subacute infective endocarditis (SBE)?**
    a. the most frequent infecting organisms (in native valves in non-intravenous (IV) drug abusers) are currently streptococci

4

b. in IV drug abusers with endocarditis, fungi are now the most common organism isolated

c. rheumatoid factor is present in 50% of patients with endocarditis of >3 weeks' duration

d. arterial sampling does not result in a better positivity than does venous sampling

e. when right-sided endocarditis occurs, the tricuspid valve is involved more commonly than the pulmonary valve

18. In a patient with a phaeochromocytoma

a. there is a 50% chance of this being familial

b. there is a 25% chance of the tumour being extra-adrenal

c. there is a 45% chance of the the tumour being malignant

d. an association with hyperthyroidism would suggest the possibility of follicular carcinoma of the thyroid

e. the diagnosis is made by estimation of vanillylmandelic acid (VMA) or metanephrine levels in a 24-h urine collection into a strong acid

19. Recognized features of hyperthyroidism due to Graves' disease include

a. thyroid-stimulating antibody (TSAb) present in >90% of cases

b. metacarpal subperiosteal new bone formation

c. hypocalcaemia

d. onycholysis

e. subnormal red cell 2,3-diphosphoglyceric acid (2,3 DPG) levels

20. Recognized clinical findings in classical mitral stenosis include

a. increased dynamic lung compliance

b. a loud first heart sound

c. a left ventricular third heart sound

d. a long diastolic murmur in severe stenosis

e. reduced perfusion of the lung bases in the upright position

21. Acyclovir

a. inhibits herpes simplex I proliferation more than herpes simplex II proliferation

b. inhibits cytomegalovirus (CMV) proliferation *in vitro* at clinically attainable concentrations

c. is rapidly phosphorylated by mammalian thymidine kinase

d. is predominantly excreted by the kidney as a phosphorylated metabolite

e. has excellent central nervous system (CNS) penetration with cerebrospinal fluid (CSF) drug levels almost identical to blood levels

22. **Which of the following are features of tabes dorsalis?**
   a. hypotonia
   b. analgesia over the nose
   c. ataxia in the absence of impaired proprioception
   d. increased gammaglobulin concentration in the CSF
   e. optic atrophy

23. **Which of the following features are consistent with a diagnosis of botulism?**
   a. strict vegetarianism
   b. fever
   c. circumoral paraesthesiae preceding muscle weakness
   d. transient improvement of muscle power by neostigmine injection
   e. extensor plantar reflexes

24. **Patients with severe thiamine deficiency**
   a. characteristically have an increased blood pyruvate level
   b. classically have a neuropathy as a consequence of demyelination
   c. are less likely to develop symptoms if maintained on a high-carbohydrate diet
   d. may be identified by demonstration of a reduced red-cell transketolase activity
   e. often experience paraesthesiae and muscle tenderness

25. **Recognized features of dystrophia myotonica include**
   a. cardiac conduction defects
   b. an abnormality of the glutamylcysteine synthetase gene which can be used to identify cases
   c. wasting of involved muscles

d. improved muscle power with testosterone therapy
e. increased catabolism of immunoglobulin G (IgG)

26. **Acute idiopathic thrombocytopenic purpura**
    a. is essentially a disease of childhood
    b. has a high mortality rate, even when treatment is prompt
    c. is associated with mucous membrane haemorrhage
    d. is improved by treatment with pooled gammaglobulin
    e. is usually treated with splenectomy

27. **Haemoglobinuria**
    a. is associated with a raised blood haptoglobin level
    b. is a sensitive sign of haemolysis
    c. occurs in blackwater fever
    d. is very common in marathon runners
    e. is a feature of congenital spherocytosis

28. **Which of the following statements about prostaglandins are true?**
    a. prostacyclin (PGI_2) inhibits platelet adhesion to vascular endothelium
    b. PGI_2 inhibits platelet degranulation
    c. PGI_2 inhibits gastric acid secretion stimulated by gastrin
    b. $PGF_{2\alpha}$ is among the most potent relaxants of pulmonary arteriolar muscle yet identified
    e. PGE_2 is a bronchodilator

29. **Primary amyloidosis**
    a. is commonly associated with a monoclonal gammopathy
    b. is characterized by amyloid protein AA deposition
    c. may be diagnosed by rectal biopsy in most cases
    d. is associated with autonomic neuropathy
    e. can be expected to regress with colchicine treatment

30. **Neurofibromatosis of the von Recklinghausen type (NF1) is associated with**
    a. meningioma in >10% of cases
    b. cutaneous pigmentation
    c. melanocytic hamartomas of the iris (Lisch nodules)
    d. phaeochromocytoma

7

e. bilateral acoustic neuromas in >5% of cases

31. Features of sickle-cell anaemia (homozygous) include
a. dactylitis
b. frontal bossing of the skull
c. abdominal pain
d. chronic leg ulceration
e. anaemia from birth

32. Which of the following are common in multiple myelomatosis?
a. a normal erythrocyte sedimentation rate (ESR)
b. pain in the skull
c. lymphadenopathy
d. back pain
e. a normal serum alkaline phosphatase level

33. The syndrome of inappropriate antidiuretic hormone (ADH) production
a. is characterized by a urine osmolality higher than the plasma osmolality
b. cannot be confidently diagnosed in the presence of hypotension
c. is a recognized complication of treatment with cisplatin
d. may be caused by demeclocycline treatment
e. is associated with osmotic demyelination syndrome

34. Polycythaemia rubra vera (PRV)
a. is usually associated with a moderately elevated ESR
b. usually terminates as an acute myeloid leukaemia
c. is associated with thrombocythaemia
d. is associated with a low leucocyte alkaline phosphatase activity
e. is associated with a prolonged bleeding time in most cases

35. Cerebral tumour
a. is likely to be found in >50% of adults first presenting with epilepsy
b. is due to metastatic tumour in the majority of cases
c. is more likely to cause epilepsy if rapidly growing

d. situated in the cerebellum, does not usually cause papilloedema except in terminal stages

e. characteristically causes positional vertigo when situated in the region of the fourth ventricle

36. **Glucose-6-phosphate dehydrogenase (G6PD) deficiency**

a. has an autosomal recessive mode of inheritance

b. may cause haemolytic anaemia in the neonate

c. is associated with defective neutrophil function only in patients with very low glucose-6-phosphate dehydrogenase activity

d. may result in haemolysis if sulphonamides are administered

e. is associated with hypoglycaemia

37. **Which of the following would be expected to follow a unilateral right hemitransection of the spinal cord at the level at which the first lumbar (L1) roots join the cord?**

a. lack of pain sensation in the left ankle

b. diminished 'two point' discrimination on the right

c. inability to determine temperature with the right foot

d. a right extensor plantar response

e. absent vibration sense at the right tibial tuberosity

38. **Which of the following features are consistent with a diagnosis of Henoch–Schönlein syndrome?**

a. a low complement C4 level

b. microscopic haematuria

c. renal IgA immune complexes

d. thrombocytopenia

e. cramping abdominal pain

39. **With regard to a rubella**

a. babies with congenital rubella are not infectious beyond the first week of life

b. administration of rubella vaccine results in a seroconversion rate of >90%

c. arthritis is a recognized feature of postnatal rubella in >50% of women

d. gammaglobulin injection in exposed pregnant women prevents viraemia

9

e. congenital rubella syndrome occurs in >50% of babies of women inadvertently vaccinated during pregnancy

40. Aminoaciduria is a feature of
a. Hartnup disease
b. Wilson's disease
c. Down's syndrome
d. severe chronic liver disease
e. galactosaemia

41. Ostium secundum atrial septal defect
a. often leads to atrial fibrillation during the second decade
b. is associated with left axis deviation on the electrocardiogram (ECG)
c. is associated with mitral valve prolapse
d. accounts for the majority of cases of atrial septal defect
e. is generally thought to require surgical correction if pulmonary blood flow is greater than twice the systemic

42. Psittacosis (ornithosis)
a. can be contracted from pigeons
b. responds to treatment with benzylpenicillin
c. is effectively excluded by a well-defined lobar pattern of consolidation on chest X-ray
d. has never been recorded to spread from person to person
e. is a cause of endocarditis

43. Features of syringomyelia with medullary extension (syringobulbia) include
a. glossopharyngeal palsy
b. Horner's syndrome
c. kyphoscoliosis
d. nystagmus
e. a narrow cervical vertebral canal

44. Congenital adrenal hyperplasia due to 21β-hydroxylase deficiency
a. is the most common variety of congenital adrenal hyperplasia
b. only occurs in females

10

c. can be treated *in utero* by administering dexamethasone to the mother to prevent virilization in affected daughters
d. is a cause of short stature
e. is associated with a salt-wasting syndrome in <50% of cases

45. Recognized features of sickle-cell trait (heterozygotes) include
a. moderate anaemia
b. reduced red-blood-cell survival
c. reduced renal concentrating ability
d. episodic haematuria
e. splenomegaly

46. Bile salts
a. are steroids
b. are excreted predominantly in conjugated form
c. deficiency is associated with reduced urinary oxylate excretion
d. are essential for medium-chain fatty acid absorption
e. in the colon inhibit water absorption

47. Systemic lupus erythematosus (SLE)
a. is not a cause of fibrinoid arterial necrosis
b. occurs equally in males and females below the age of 30 years
c. is associated with proteinuria in <50% of cases of significant renal disease
d. is associated with lymphadenopathy during disease exacerbations
e. is associated with joint symptoms in <30% of cases

48. Which of the following support a diagnosis of primary hyperaldosteronism (Conn's syndrome) due to an adrenal adenoma?
a. muscle weakness
b. hypertension
c. high blood renin levels
d. hyperkalaemia
e. fall of plasma aldosterone levels on standing

11

49. **Pseudohypoparathyroidism (PHP) type I (of the type associated with somatic abnormality)**
   a. is a congenital disorder
   b. is associated with markedly increased urinary cAMP excretion in response to exogenous parathyroid hormone administration
   c. is a cause of hyperphosphataemia
   d. is usually associated with a normal serum calcium
   e. responds to parathyroid hormone (PTH) administration

50. **Vitamin B_{12} deficiency may result in**
   a. sensory ataxia
   b. optic neuritis
   c. psychosis
   d. 'glove-and-stocking' anaesthesia
   e. increased urinary methylmalonyl CoA excretion

51. **Recognized features of vitamin D deficiency include**
   a. craniosynostosis
   b. hypophosphataemia
   c. growth retardation
   d. proximal muscle weakness
   e. increased serum alkaline phosphatase activity

52. **β-Thalassaemia major (homozygous)**
   a. is characterized by persistence of fetal haemoglobin (HbF)
   b. is associated with a chronic marked reticulocytosis
   c. is always associated with a raised proportion of HbA_2
   d. is very rarely associated with circulating nucleated red cells
   e. is a cause of pathological fracture of long bones

53. **Features consistent with a diagnosis of chronic primary autoimmune adrenal insufficiency include**
   a. microcytic hypochromic anaemia
   b. hyperpigmentation of mucous membranes
   c. anorexia
   d. diabetes mellitus
   e. orthostatic hypotension

54. The phrenic nerve
a. arises predominantly from the third cervical nerve
b. is a purely motor nerve
c. enters the thorax lying on the lateral aspect of the vertebrae
d. runs in front of the root of the lung
e. innervates the diaphragm from below

55. In acromegaly
a. circulating insulin-like growth factor (IGF-I) levels are characteristically low
b. hypoadrenocorticism is associated in >50% of cases
c. hypertriglyceridaemia occurs as a consequence of reduced lipoprotein lipase activity
d. 1,25-hydroxycholecalciferol levels are increased
e. prolactin levels are increased in up to 40% of cases

56. Hyperlipidaemia occurring in long-standing cholestasis
a. is associated with increased lecithin cholesterol acyl transferase (LCAT) activity
b. is associated with accelerated development of atheroma
c. is characteristically associated with tendinous xanthomas
d. is characteristically associated with palmar xanthomas
e. is characterized by an increased level of circulating free cholesterol

57. As regards herpes simplex encephalitis
a. it is usually due to herpes simplex virus type 1 (HSV1) infection
b. >80% of cases are in patients aged <10 years
c. herpes labialis precedes encephalitis in >30% of cases
d. it is associated with the development of focal neurological signs in most patients
e. it is not increased in frequency in patients who are immunocompromised

58. Causes of raised serum conjugated bilirubin levels, with relatively normal serum transaminase levels, include
a. primary biliary cirrhosis
b. viral hepatitis

c. the Dubin–Johnson syndrome
d. testosterone therapy
e. Gilbert's syndrome

59. **Features of Gaucher's disease (glucocerebrosidase deficiency) include**
a. great enlargement of the spleen
b. a cherry-red macular spot
c. areas of decalcification in bones
d. raised serum, tartrate-labile, acid phosphatase activity
e. accumulation of sphingomyelin in various tissues

60. **Ascites complicating cirrhosis is**
a. most commonly infected by anaerobic Gram-negative bacteria when spontaneous peritonitis develops
b. associated with an increased ANF level
c. usually associated with a small isolated left-sided pleural effusion
d. characterized by a protein level of >20 g/l in the peritoneal fluid
e. associated with decreased renin levels

61. **Chronic active autoimmune hepatitis**
a. usually presents as an acute hepatitis
b. rarely presents before 20 years of age
c. is associated with cytotoxic/suppressor T-cell (OKT-3) infiltration of the portal region on liver histology
d. is associated with hypogammaglobulinaemia
e. is rarely associated with antinuclear antibody (ANA)

62. **Primary biliary cirrhosis**
a. is associated with the presence of mitochondrial antibodies in the serum in <75% of cases
b. is often associated with the sicca syndrome
c. usually presents with progressive jaundice; rarely pruritus may precede the onset of jaundice
d. is commonly associated with enlarged nodes in the porta hepatis
e. affects females in 90% of cases

14

63. **Features of hereditary haemorrhagic telangiectasia include**
   a. gastrointestinal haemorrhage as the usual presenting feature
   b. pulmonary arteriovenous malformations
   c. telangiectasia of the mucous membranes, but not on the skin
   d. tendency of lesions to become less obvious with age
   e. a therapeutic response to oestrogens

64. **Features of homocystinuria (cystathionine β-synthetase deficiency) include**
   a. arachnodactyly
   b. generalized osteoporosis
   c. venous thromboses
   d. arterial thromboses
   e. a clinical response to pyridoxine

65. **Which of the following would be expected findings in a recently diagnosed patient aged 20 years with insulin-dependent diabetes mellitus? (IDDM)**
   a. circulating cytoplasmic islet cell antibodies (ICA)
   b. insulin autoantibodies (IAA)
   c. antibodies to the 64KDa antigen (glutamic acid decarboxylase, GAD)
   d. human leucocyte antigen (HLA)-DR3 or HLA-DR4-positive
   e. increased HbA_{1c} levels

66. **Hepatitis C virus (HCV)**
   a. is less infectious than hepatitis B (HBV)
   b. is inactivated by heat treatment of blood
   c. causes jaundice in >50% of those infected
   d. results in chronic hepatitis in >40% of those infected
   e. usually responds to interferon treatment (as reflected by reduced transaminase levels)

67. **Recognized features of abetalipoproteinaemia include**
   a. high serum cholesterol concentration
   b. palmar xanthomas
   c. advanced atherosclerotic vascular disease
   d. abnormal red blood cell morphology
   e. severe mental retardation

68. **Glycosuria may occur**
  a. in association with acromegaly
  b. in association with subarachnoid haemorrhage
  c. in association with phaeochromocytoma
  d. as a result of anxiety
  e. as a complication of gastrectomy

69. **Recognized features of idiopathic hypoparathyroidism include**
  a. increased urinary phosphate excretion in response to PTH injection
  b. increased urinary calcium excretion
  c. convulsions
  d. tetany
  e. a familial history in most cases

70. **With respect to intravenous thrombolytic therapy for myocardial infarction, which of the following statements are correct?**
  a. recombinant tissue plasminogen activator (rt-PA) more rapidly results in arterial recannulation than does streptokinase
  b. the benefit of streptokinase is enhanced by combination with aspirin
  c. streptokinase when administered within 6 h is just as effective as when administered within 2 h of the onset of symptoms
  d. in patients administered streptokinase, ventricular fibrillation is more frequent than in controls
  e. streptokinase has a more profound effect on mortality in the case of small infarcts than in the case of larger infarcts

71. **Systemic sclerosis (scleroderma)**
  a. generally has a better prognosis if Raynaud's syndrome is not a feature
  b. with impending renal deterioration can usually be predicted by identification of raised renin levels
  c. is associated with telangiectasia which classically has no central arteriole

16

d. associated with anticentromere antibody is associated with a better prognosis than cases where the antibody is not present
e. is associated with normal radiological oesophageal abnormality in >40% of cases

72. **Individuals with porphobilinogen (PBG) deaminase deficiency (the basis of acute intermittent porphyria)**
a. have markedly increased faecal protoporphyrin excretion during attacks
b. excrete excessive urinary PBG between acute attacks
c. have a greater than 75% chance of remaining asymptomatic throughout their lives
d. experience significant photosensitivity
e. who manifest clinical disease generally present within the first decade of life

73. **Recognized features of giant-cell arteritis include**
a. absent temporal arterial pulsation
b. associated symptoms and signs of polymyalgia rheumatica in >30% of cases
c. granulomatous arteritis demonstrable in most cases on temporal artery biopsy
d. an unelevated ESR in 20% of cases
e. a requirement for long-term steroid treatment (>3 years) in <33% of cases

74. **Which of the following drugs are considered safe to give to a patient known to have acute intermittent porphyria?**
a. suxamethonium
b. carbamazepine
c. sulphonamide
d. penicillin
e. morphine

75. **Features of Bartter's syndrome include**
a. hypokalaemic alkalosis
b. aldosterone deficiency
c. elevated plasma renin activity

17

d. resistance to the effect of infused angiotensin

e. atrophy of the juxtaglomerular apparatus

76. Which of the following features is inconsistent with a diagnosis of diabetic nephropathy?

a. expansion of the glomerular mesangial matrix on renal biopsy

b. exercise-induced microalbuminaemia

c. nephrotic syndrome

d. red-cell casts in the urinary sediment

e. the absence of retinopathy

77. The Philadelphia chromosome

a. represents an additional long arm of chromosome 22

b. is associated with a better prognosis when it is present in chronic myeloid leukaemia (CML) than when it is not present

c. is found in >40% of cases of myelofibrosis

d. is present in both myeloid and erythroid lines in CML

e. is found in >10% of cases of acute lymphoblastic leukaemia in adults

78. Which of the following features seen in the urinary sediment usually indicate significant renal pathology?

a. hyaline casts

b. epithelial-cell casts

c. large wide casts

d. epithelial cells

e. white-cell casts

79. Clinical features of VP include

a. increased skin fragility

b. hypertrichosis

c. skin pigmentation

d. acute neurological attacks

e. increased faecal porphyrin excretion

80. With respect to the carcinoid syndrome

a. 40% of cases are associated with a bronchial tumour

b. carcinoid syndrome occurs more commonly as a

complication of hindgut tumours than of small-bowel
tumours

c. hypokalaemia, hypercalcaemia and metabolic acidosis
suggest a vasoactive intestinal peptide (VIP)-secreting tumour
rather than carcinoid

d. circulating chromogranin A is associated only with a
minority of advanced carcinoid tumours

e. patients with foregut carcinoids often excrete urine
containing relatively little 5-hydroxyindoleacetic acid but
large amounts of 5-hydroxytryptophan

81. **Recognized features of tetralogy of Fallot include**
a. a loud pulmonary second sound
b. absence of cyanosis at 6 months of age
c. cyanosis improved by mild exercise
d. clubbing at birth
e. right bundle branch block on the ECG

82. **With respect to bone marrow transplantation**
a. allogeneic or syngeneic bone marrow transplantation is
capable of producing a 5-year disease-free survival in >50%
of cases of CML transplanted in the chronic phase

b. patients transplanted from related donors with one human
leucocyte antigen (HLA) A, B or D locus mismatch have a
significantly worse survival than do HLA-identical sibling
transplants

c. a lower rate of relapse of leukaemia occurs in patients who
develop acute or chronic graft-versus-host disease (GvHD)

d. <10% of patients receiving marrow transplants from HLA-
identical siblings develop significant acute GvHD

e. almost all patients with chronic GvHD will require
indefinite treatment with prednisolone (with or without
cyclosporin)

83. **Features favouring a diagnosis of ectopic
adrenocorticotrophic hormone (ACTH) syndrome rather
than an ACTH-secreting pituitary tumour (Cushing's
disease) include**
a. a florid cushingoid appearance
b. hypokalaemia

    c. very high unstimulated circulating ACTH levels
    d. an increased ACTH production response to stimulation with corticotrophin releasing hormone (CRH)
    e. suppression of plasma cortisol by dexamethasone

84. **Psoriasis**
    a. is usually an itchy eruption
    b. exhibits the Kobner phenomenon
    c. predominantly affects the flexor surfaces
    d. is associated with hyperuricaemia
    e. of the guttate variety is less likely to pursue a chronic course than is the case with other presentations of psoriasis

85. **Lichen planus**
    a. never itches
    b. frequently involves the genital area
    c. may affect the nails
    d. is characterized by papular skin lesions
    e. may leave residual pigmentation after resolution

86. **Which of the following skin lesions are associated with internal malignancy?**
    a. necrobiosis lipoidica
    b. granuloma annulare
    c. necrolytic migratory erythema
    d. acquired ichthyosis
    e. erythema gyratum repens

87. **A diagnosis of tuberculoid, rather than lepromatous, leprosy is favoured by**
    a. acid-fast bacilli in the skin smear
    b. depressed cell-mediated immunity
    c. a negative lepromin test
    d. anaesthetic skin lesions
    e. symmetrical 'glove-and-stocking' anaesthesia

88. **Which of the following are uricosuric in usual therapeutic dosage?**
    a. ethacrynic acid
    b. allopurinol

c. pyrazinamide
d. sulphinpyrazone
e. probenecid

89. **Features of haemophilia A (congenital factor VIII deficiency) include**
a. the identification of female carriers by DNA probe in >90% of cases
b. antifactor VIII antibodies are identified in >75% of cases
c. a normal antigenic factor VIIIc level
d. a prolonged PT
e. no family history (new mutation) in >25% of cases

90. **Which of the following are true statements with respect to minimal-change nephrotic syndrome (MCNS)?**
a. serum IgG levels are usually reduced in MCNS
b. macroscopic haematuria occurs in 30% of cases of MCNS
c. MCNS is associated with disruption of the glomerular basement membrane
d. MCNS is usually accompanied by a low serum C3 complement level
e. in children MCNS rarely results in a serum albumin level below 30 g/l

91. **Electrocardiographic findings of the Wolff–Parkinson–White syndrome include**
a. a QRS interval of longer than 0.11 s
b. a predominant R wave in lead Vi
c. T-wave inversion in lead aVL
d. deep Q waves in lead III
e. δ waves

92. **Extensor plantar reflexes with absent knee jerks may occur in**
a. spinal cord compression at the third and fourth lumbar levels
b. Friedreich's ataxia
c. pernicious anaemia
d. multiple sclerosis
e. taboparesis

93. **Clinical features consistent with a diagnosis of Friedreich's ataxia include**
a. a positive Romberg test
b. delayed latency on visual evoked potential testing
c. widespread T-wave inversion on ECG
d. extensor plantar reflexes
e. axonal sensory neuropathy demonstrated on electrophysiology

94. **Recognized features of coeliac disease include**
a. a protein-losing enteropathy
b. an association with the B27 tissue type
c. associated disaccharidase deficiency
d. interstitial hypermobility
e. skin hyperpigmentation

95. **There is a recognized association between cataract and**
a. dystrophia myotonica
b. scleroderma (systemic sclerosis)
c. galactosaemia
d. Down's syndrome
e. Hurler's syndrome

96. **Corticosteroids are of established therapeutic benefit in**
a. Gilbert's syndrome
b. primary biliary cirrhosis
c. chronic active hepatitis
d. prolonged cholestasis following viral hepatitis A
e. acute hepatic failure

97. **The ECG in hyperkalaemia classically shows**
a. a shortened PR interval
b. prominent U waves
c. inverted T waves
d. increased R-wave amplitude
e. increased QRS duration

98. **Recognized causes of generalized pruritus include**
a. scabies
b. haemolytic jaundice

22

c. myxoedema
d. secondary syphilis
e. Hodgkin's disease

99. **In motor neuron disease (MND)**
   a. electromyography reveals fibrillation potentials
   b. there is atrophy of the Betz cells of the motor cortex
   c. there is no sensory impairment
   d. nerve conduction velocity is usually reduced
   e. plantar reflexes are generally flexor

100. **A positive (orange) reaction when the urine is tested by the Clinitest method may occur in association with**
   a. alkaptonuria
   b. galactosaemia
   c. salicylate therapy
   d. isoniazid therapy
   e. ascorbic acid consumption

101. **Rheumatic fever**
   a. is commonly associated with carditis when it affects young children
   b. is more likely to occur in a patient who develops nephritis following a streptococcal infection
   c. is likely to occur in about one in 30 people who develop pharyngitis caused by a rheumatogenic strain of streptococci during an epidemic
   d. is unlikely to reccur in a patient who previously developed rheumatic fever on re-exposure to a rheumatogenic strain of streptococci since he or she will have developed an antibody response
   e. is associated with a progressively rising antistreptolysin-O (ASO) titre in severe cases

102. **In classical osteogenesis imperfecta (OI; type III)**
   a. fractures occur *in utero*
   b. the teeth are usually normal
   c. blue sclerae generally become more obvious with age
   d. there is an increased incidence of osteosarcoma
   e. the long bones are excessively radiopaque on X-ray

23

103. **Psoriatic arthropathy**
   a. is supported by the finding of a total of six nail pits
   b. tends to cause a more symmetrical arthritis than is the case with rheumatoid arthritis
   c. is rarely (<5% of cases) associated with sacroiliitis
   d. is associated with iritis in >25% of cases
   e. is a recognized complication of acquired immunodeficiency syndrome (AIDS)

104. **Short stature is a characteristic feature of**
   a. cirrhosis in childhood
   b. homocystinuria
   c. Hurler's syndrome
   d. chronic renal failure in childhood
   e. pseudohypoparathyroidism

105. **Attacks of hypoglycaemia are a recognized complication of**
   a. von Gierke's disease
   b. galactosaemia
   c. G6PD deficiency
   d. fructosaemia
   e. Gaucher's disease

106. **Features consistent with a diagnosis of Tay–Sachs disease include**
   a. neonatal hypotonicity
   b. hepatomegaly
   c. significantly reduced head circumference at 2 years
   d. convulsions
   e. cerebral syringomyelin accumulation

107. **Felty's syndrome**
   a. is more common in patients with IgM rheumatoid factor seronegative rheumatoid arthritis
   b. is characteristically associated with hypogammaglobulinaemia
   c. is haematologically improved by splenectomy in >50% of cases
   d. is usually associated with myeloid hypoplasia on marrow examination

e. spontaneously remits within 12 months in most (>60%) patients

108. With respect to interferon
a. α-interferon (IFN-α) is predominantly synthesized by fibroblasts
b. interferons exert cellular effects by virtue of interaction with specific receptors
c. γ-interferon (IFN-γ) synthesis by T cells occurs in response to viral infection
d. IFN-γ is a major activator of macrophages
e. IFN-α is effective in chronic hepatitis C

109. An insulinoma
a. has a recognized association with hypercalcaemia
b. is solitary in >80% of cases
c. leads to hypoglycaemia after prolonged fast (48 h) in most cases (>90%)
d. is usually associated with a raised insulin : proinsulin ratio
e. would be expected to release insulin after tolbutamide administration

110. With reference to interleukins
a. IL-6 is the most important factor stimulating IL-1 release
b. IL-2 receptors are not present on resting (unstimulated) T cells
c. IL-1 stimulates C-reactive protein synthesis
d. activation of T cells causes release of IL-2
e. IL-6 is a mediator of T-cell stimulation of B-cell proliferation

111. Herpes zoster
a. is localized to one or two dermatomes and identification of additional vesicles at more distant sites excludes the diagnosis
b. more frequently involves the ophthalmic than the maxillary branch of the trigeminal nerves
c. is a cause of facial paralysis
d. is a cause of encephalomyelitis
e. is an untenable diagnosis if there is tender lymphadenopathy of the regional lymph nodes shortly after the development of the rash

112. **Whooping cough (pertussis)**
   a. infectivity is not reduced by erythromycin treatment
   b. almost never occurs in adults who have been vaccinated as children
   c. is characteristically associated with a polymorph leucocytosis
   d. is associated with convulsions less frequently than is the case with other febrile conditions
   e. rapidly resolves with ampicillin treatment

113. **With which of the following conditions is intracerebral calcification associated?**
   a. congenital toxoplasmosis
   b. glioblastoma multiforme
   c. cysticercosis
   d. tuberose sclerosis
   e. oliogodendroglioma

114. **A short PR interval of the ECG is associated with**
   a. hypertrophic obstructive cardiomyopathy (HOCM)
   b. dystrophia myotonica
   c. the Lown–Ganong–Levine syndrome
   d. rheumatic carditis
   e. Duchenne muscular dystrophy

115. **Accepted features of niacin deficiency include**
   a. peripheral neuropathy
   b. glossitis
   c. dermatitis
   d. depression
   e. congestive cardiac failure

116. **Findings consistent with a diagnosis of Hurler's syndrome in a child aged 2 years include**
   a. joint hypermobility
   b. short extremities
   c. a normal IQ
   d. cataract
   e. splenomegaly

117. **In severe hepatocellular liver disease**
   a. blood factor VIII levels are usually reduced
   b. the bleeding diathesis is due to deficient coagulation factors and cannot be effectively reversed by administration of banked blood
   c. blood factor VII levels are usually reduced
   d. spur cells in the blood film indicate a poor prognosis
   e. it is safe to perform a percutaneous liver biopsy unless the patient's PT is >15 s longer than the control

118. **Infectious mononucleosis**
   a. is often asymptomatic in children
   b. is associated with lymphadenopathy in <50% of teenagers who have clinical infection
   c. is associated with heterophile antibody which is absorbed by guinea-pig kidney
   d. is rarely associated with abnormal tests of liver function
   e. is associated with autoimmune heamolytic anaemia, usually of the cold agglutinin, IgM type

119. **A Mendelian X-linked dominant condition would be expected to be transmitted to**
   a. half of the daughters of an affected woman
   b. all of the sons of an affected woman
   c. all children of an affected man
   d. half of the sons of an affected woman
   e. all daughters of an affected man

120. **Cutaneous anthrax**
   a. causes a black eschar which overlies pus
   b. lesions are usually painful and tender
   c. lesions are associated with marked oedema
   d. has a mortality of about 20%, even when antibiotics are given
   e. is very likely to occur in people exposed to anthrax spores

121. **Pyogenic meningitis**
   a. in adults is more commonly a result of pneumococcal than meningococcal infection

b. is most commonly due to *Haemophilus influenzae* in a 3-year-old child

c. due to *H. influenzae* is more likely to be complicated by subdural effusions than that due to *Streptococcus pneumoniae*

d. due to Gram-negative bacteria (excluding *H. influenzae*) is most frequently due to *Escherichia coli*

e. due to meningococcus can be identified in the CSF by Gram stain in >50% of cases in which it is subsequently grown

122. In diffuse fibrotic lung disease
a. the forced expiratory volume in 1 s/forced vital capacity (FEV_1/FVC) ratio is usually decreased
b. the arterial Pco_2 is classically increased
c. there is generally significant ventilation–perfusion inequality
d. reduction of single-breath carbon monoxide transfer is an early feature
e. gallium scanning generally shows decreased pulmonary uptake

123. Which of the following statements are true?
a. the ascending limb of the loop of Henle is highly permeable to water
b. intraluminal fluid entering the distal convoluted tubule is hypertonic with respect to the surrounding extracellular fluid
c. arginine vasopressin (AVP) reduces the permeability of the distal convoluted tubule to water
d. there is active transport of Na^+ out of the descending limb of the loop of Henle
e. approximately 20% of the glomerular filtrate is reabsorbed into the proximal tubule of the nephron

124. Characteristic features of constrictive pericarditis include
a. cardiac failure without serious dyspnoea
b. a sharp y descent of the jugular venous pressure
c. a pericardial knock (palpable third heart sound)
d. an inspiratory rise of the jugular venous pressure
e. a fall of the systemic arterial pressure during inspiration

125. Which of the following conditions are associated with dissecting aneurysm of the aorta?
a. syphilitic aortitis

b. coarctation of the aorta

c. hypertension

d. Marfan's syndrome

e. homocystinuria

126. **Splitting of the second heart sound**

   a. is increased in pulmonary valve stenosis

   b. is increased when right bundle branch block occurs

   c. is reversed in the presence of left bundle branch block

   d. is increased in the presence of uncomplicated pulmonary hypertension

   e. is increased during expiration

127. **There is an increased risk of developing carcinoma of the large bowel in**

   a. Gardner's syndrome

   b. ulcerative colitis

   c. Ménétrier's disease

   d. familial colonic polyposis

   e. pre-existing colonic adenomas

128. **Which of the following support a diagnosis of leptospirosis?**

   a. leucopenia

   b. myalgia

   c. thrombocytopenia

   d. meningism

   e. conjunctivitis

129. **There is a recognized association between hyperuricaemia and**

   a. type I glycogen storage disease (von Gierke's disease)

   b. Down's syndrome

   c. starvation

   d. xanthinuria

   e. psoriasis

130. **Reiter's syndrome**

   a. is more commonly associated with keratoderma blenorrhagica when it follows chlamidial urethritis than when bacillary dysentry is the cause

b. is more commonly seen in females
c. is associated with the HLA B27 tissue type
d. may be associated with urethritis when it follows an attack of dysentery
e. responds to specific antimicrobial therapy when it follows bacillary dysentry

131. Chronic lymphatic leukaemia (CLL)
a. may transform into a diffuse histiocytic lymphoma (immunoblastic lymphoma)
b. is the commonest form of leukaemia seen in the elderly in the UK
c. is associated with vesiculobullous skin lesions
d. is associated with a monoclonal band on electrophoresis in <10% of cases
e. terminates as acute leukaemia in about 25% of cases

132. Drug-induced lupus erythematosus syndrome
a. is frequently associated with proteinuria
b. is usually associated with antibodies to Sm
c. is not usually associated with the presence of lupus erythematosus-cells
d. is usually associated with a normal serum complement (C3) level
e. occurs in females more than twice as frequently as in males

133. Lyme disease
a. is usually transmitted to humans by mosquito bites
b. is associated with a characteristic erythema marginatum rash
c. is a cause of lymphocytic meningitis
d. is caused by a *Mycoplasma*-type organism
e. is reliably and rapidly treated by penicillin

134. Ankylosing spondylitis
a. is associated with iritis attacks which are usually bilateral
b. presents as a peripheral arthritis in >50% of cases
c. predisposes to fracture of the cervical spine in advanced cases
d. can be predicted to develop in >60% of asymptomatic people identified to be HLA B27-positive
e. is now recognized to occur equally in males and females

135. **Vascular 'spider' telangiectasia in association with liver disease**
   a. is usually most numerous over the abdomen
   b. does not blanch on pressure
   c. always persists, even when hepatic function improves
   d. may be pulsatile
   e. results from dilation of venules

136. **Infection by *Cryptococcus neoformans* involving the CNS**
   a. is limited in the CSF since *Cryptococcus* activates the alternative complement pathway
   b. is associated with a moderately increased white-cell count with a predominance of lymphocytes
   c. is associated with cranial nerve lesions
   d. commonly presents with seizures
   e. is usually associated with marked neck rigidity

137. **The Zollinger–Ellison syndrome**
   a. is diagnosed by the demonstration of raised gastrin levels and achlorhydria
   b. is associated with excessive gastrin secretion after calcium infusion
   c. more commonly results from primary antral G-cell hyperplasia than a pancreatic adenoma
   d. is associated with hyperparathyroidism
   e. results in gastric mucosal hypertrophy

138. **Migraine**
   a. may cause a hemianopia which persists for 12 h
   b. headache tends to be aggravated by straining
   c. may be complicated by ophthalmoplegia
   d. may be complicated by Horner's syndrome
   e. usually becomes increasingly severe with age

139. **Tamoxifen treatment**
   a. is associated in tumour regression in over 50% of unselected patients with metastatic breast carcinoma
   b. is equally likely to be associated with tumour regression in postmenopausal patients who are oestrogen receptor (ER)-negative as in those who are ER-positive

31

c. is more likely to result in success in patients who have tumours which have both progesterone receptors (PGR) and ERs than in those who have ER receptors but are PGR-negative
d. generally results in longer periods of remission in responsive patients who are ER-positive than in those who are ER-negative
e. suppresses ovulation in over 95% of premenopausal patients

140. **Which of the following are recognized features of mumps infection?**
a. lymphocytic meningitis
b. purulent discharge from the parotid duct
c. clinical orchitis in <25% of adult males who become infected
d. subclinical infection in >25% of cases
e. a higher incidence in the first year of life and more severe disease than in the second year

141. **In patients with chronic renal disease due to analgesic nephropathy**
a. it is almost always associated with a reduction of urinary concentrating ability
b. the glomerular filtration rate is generally normal even in the presence of moderate uraemia
c. nephrotic syndrome occurs in 20%
d. there is an increased risk of developing transitional cell carcinomas of the uroepithelium
e. microscopic haematuria is usually due to a transitional cell carcinoma

142. **Recognized features of paracetamol poisoning include**
a. methaemoglobinaemia
b. early onset of coma
c. acute renal failure
d. hyperventilation during the first 24 h after ingestion
e. prolonged PT

143. **Varicella**
a. tends to be a milder disease in adults than in children
b. never causes lesions on the palms of the hands

c. causes lesions which occur in the mouth
d. causes lesions which do not occur in crops
e. is usually associated with a 3–4-day prodromal period

144. Infectious hepatitis (hepatitis A)
a. has a longer incubation period than hepatitis B (serum hepatitis)
b. is usually spread by the faecal–oral route
c. is not infectious until 3–4 days after the onset of jaundice
d. is a cause of fulminant hepatic failure
e. is usually resolving 2 weeks after the onset of illness

145. Hypercalcaemia is associated with
a. lithium therapy
b. secondary hyperparathyroidism
c. excessive absorbable alkali consumption
d. sarcoidosis
e. acute adrenal failure

146. Rabies
a. is an RNA virus
b. virus persists in the bones of dead animals for long periods after death from rabies
c. has a long incubation period of usually >4 months
d. does not occur in cats
e. virus can penetrate unbroken skin

147. Dietary deficiency of iron resulting in anaemia
a. is more likely in patients with achlorhydria than in those with normal gastric acidity
b. is associated with a reduced overall mean corpuscular haemoglobin (MCH) value
c. is commonly associated with anisocytosis in the early stages
d. is generally associated with a reduced reticulocyte count
e. is associated with increased serum ferritin levels

148. Recognized features of cystic fibrosis include
a. decreased sweat sodium concentrate in response to aldosterone administration

b. nasal polyposis
c. hepatic portal fibrosis
d. aspermia
e. albumin in the stool

149. **Clinical signs consistent with lobar consolidation include**
   a. reduced chest movement
   b. whispering pectoriloquy
   c. a pleural rub
   d. diminished vocal fremitus
   e. deviation of the trachea

150. **Acute idiopathic polyneuritis (Guillain–Barré syndrome) is characteristically associated with**
   a. an increased number of polymorphonuclear white cells in the CSF
   b. paraesthesiae of the toes as the first neurological symptom in most cases
   c. early loss of tendon reflexes
   d. almost invariable demonstration of reduced nerve conduction velocity in cases with motor weakness
   e. a CSF protein of <20 g/l

151. **Results of acclimatization to the hypoxia of altitude include**
   a. a decreased affinity of haemoglobin for oxygen
   b. a reduced $Paco_2$ level
   c. a decreased ventilatory response to carbon dioxide
   d. a shift to the left of the oxygen dissociation curve
   e. decreased red-cell 2,3 DPG concentration

152. ***Mycoplasma pneumoniae***
   a. infection is associated with the development of agglutinins to a non-haemolytic streptococcus
   b. can be grown on a cell-free medium
   c. predominantly causes infection in the elderly
   d. infection is associated with a polymorphonuclear leucocytosis
   e. infection is associated with the development of the Stevens–Johnson syndrome

34

153. **Which of the following statements relating to immunoglobulin are true?**
   a. papain cleavage produces two heavy and two light chains
   b. heavy chains do not have 'variable' regions
   c. IgM does not cross the placenta
   d. antigen-bound IgM activates complement
   e. κ chains are heavy chains

154. **Which of the following are true statements with respect to the CSF?**
   a. sodium concentration is lower than in the plasma
   b. the albumin:globulin ratio is 8 : 1
   c. the chloride concentration is lower than in the plasma
   d. the pH is identical to the plasma pH
   e. the glucose concentration is higher than in the plasma

155. **Aldosterone**
   a. is produced by the juxtaglomerular apparatus
   b. acts predominantly on the proximal convoluted tubule
   c. inhibits water resorption
   d. causes increased urinary sodium excretion
   e. dependent urinary potassium loss is uninfluenced by reduction of sodium intake

156. **Antineutrophil cytoplasmic antibodies (ANCAs)**
   a. are found in most patients with Wegener's granulomatosis
   b. are common in classical polyarteritis nodosa
   c. are likely to be found in cases of severe focal proliferative glomerulonephritis
   d. titres tend to be related to disease activity
   e. with a diffuse cytoplasmic pattern are characteristic of Wegener's granulomatosis

157. **α-Adrenergic sympathetic stimulation results in**
   a. decreased insulin secretion in response to a glucose load
   b. axillary sweating
   c. bronchoconstriction
   d. lipolysis
   e. vasodilation

158. **Results of prolonged severe vomiting complicating pyloric stenosis include**
   a. hyperchloraemia
   b. impaired renal bicarbonate excretion
   c. hypoventilation
   d. acidic urine excretion
   e. hypokalaemia

159. **With regard to atrial myxoma**
   a. myxomas are the commonest primary cardiac tumours
   b. the mean age for diagnosis of sporadic myxoma is 30 years
   c. sporadic myxoma is more common in females
   d. slightly more myxomas occur in the left atrium than the right atrium
   e. in over 30% of cases multiple tumours are present

160. **With regard to peripheral nerve damage**
   a. fibrillation potentials are not characteristic in neuropraxia
   b. immediately after total transection of the nerve, marked fibrillation potentials are observed in the innervated muscle
   c. sensory action potentials tend to be preserved in root lesions
   d. evoked sensory or motor action potentials are characteristically reduced in axonal neuropathies
   e. conduction velocity is markedly delayed in neuropathies in which demyelination is prominent

161. **Two months after splenectomy for traumatic rupture of the spleen what findings are expected on examination of the peripheral blood film?**
   a. target cells
   b. Heinz bodies
   c. Howell–Jolly bodies
   d. anisocytosis
   e. numerous nucleated red cells

162. **Which of the following diagnostic features are consistent with a diagnosis of toxic shock syndrome (TSS)?**
   a. circulating antibody to the TSST-1 toxin
   b. temperature of 41°C
   c. a serum creatine phosphokinase of 20 000 u/l

d. mucosal membrane hyperaemia

e. a serum alanine serum transferase (AST) of
80 i.u./l (normal range <35 i.u./l)

163. Following subarachnoid rupture of a cerebral aneurysm

a. hydrocephalus would be expected to occur in about 10% of cases

b. computed tomographic scan on the first day will show intracranial blood in over 90% of cases

c. xanthochromia of the CSF would still be an expected finding 2 days after haemorrhage

d. papilloedema occurs in >30% of cases

e. there is more chance of rebleeding than is the case with vascular malformations

164. With which of the following conditions are target cells associated?

a. autoimmune haemolytic anaemia

b. haemoglobin C disease

c. iron deficiency

d. thalassaemia minor (heterozygous)

e. sideroblastic anaemia

165. Immunoglobulin A deficiency

a. is much less common than IgG deficiency

b. is associated with increased rates of antibody to milk protein

c. is frequently associated with the development of antibodies to IgA

d. is associated with duodenal ulceration

e. is frequently found in patients with ataxia telangiectasia

166. A lesion

a. at the left optic radiation results in a homonymous hemianopia

b. of the optic tract results in unilateral blindness

c. at the level of the chiasma, due to pituitary tumour, may result in a homonymous hemianopia

d. in the temporal lobe may result in a lower quadrantic homonymous anopia

e. of the visual cortex results in a homonymous field defect, which is always congruous

167. **The facial nerve**
   a. originates from a nucleus in the medulla
   b. runs a course round the fourth nucleus in the brainstem
   c. runs in the cerebellopontine angle
   d. is the motor nerve to the stapedius muscle
   e. conveys gustatory sensory fibres in the upper stylomastoid canal

168. **Results of division of the common peroneal nerve, at the level of the upper fibula, include**
   a. loss of power to evert the foot
   b. decreased sensation over the dorsum of the foot
   c. loss of plantar flexion at the ankle joint
   d. wasting of tibialis anterior
   e. loss of the plantar reflex

169. **A patient with autosomal dominant polycystic kidney disease**
   a. has a 50% chance of progressing to end-stage renal failure
   b. has a 90% chance of one or more family members having multiple cysts on abdominal ultrasound
   c. can be diagnosed using genetic probes to genes linked to autosomal dominant polycystic kidney disease (ADPKD)-1
   d. is associated with urinary calculi in up to 30% of cases
   e. is unlikely to complain of abdominal distension and bloating associated with the disease

170. **Wegener's granulomatosis**
   a. is most commonly associated with a rapidly progressive focal necrotizing GN when there is renal involvement
   b. is usually (in >80% of cases) associated with the finding of ANCAs, with the characteristic diffuse cytoplasmic staining (C-ANCA)
   c. disease activity can be monitored, in most cases where it is present, by ANCAs

d. survival has been significantly increased by steroid use but addition of cyclophosphamide improves this to a small extent
e. is excluded by the finding of diffuse proliferative glomerulonephritis on renal biopsy

171. *Schistosoma haematobium*
  a. infection is endemic in the Indian subcontinent
  b. eggs excite a local granulomatous tissue reaction
  c. worms colonize the mesenteric veins
  d. eggs have a lateral spine
  e. eggs are excreted in the urine

172. **After intravenous injection of secretin (1 i.u./kg) classical findings on duodenal sampling include**
  a. a high enzyme concentration in chronic pancreatitis
  b. a low bicarbonate concentration in chronic pancreatitis
  c. a low volume in cystic fibrosis
  d. an absent rise in the volume of pancreatic secretion after vagotomy has been performed
  e. a normal bicarbonate concentration when a carcinoma partially obstructs the pancreatic duct

173. **Secretin**
  a. release is inhibited by somatostatin
  b. stimulates pancreatic bicarbonate secretion
  c. enhances the secretion of pancreatic enzymes in response to vagal stimulation
  d. is secreted in response to glucose perfusion of the duodenum
  e. results in a reduction of lower oesophageal sphincter tone only at pharmacological levels

174. **Cholecystokinin**
  a. is produced and secreted by the gastric antral mucosa
  b. regulates concentration of bile in the gallbladder
  c. causes contraction of the sphincter of Oddi
  d. stimulates pancreatic enzyme secretion
  e. stimulates bowel mobility

175. **Bronchopulmonary aspergillosis**
  a. occurs predominantly in summer months

b. is often associated with segmental collapse
c. is associated with specific precipitating IgG antibodies
d. is diagnosed by culture of *Aspergillus fumigatus* from the sputum
e. is associated with fever

176. **African visceral leishmaniasis (kala-azar)**
a. is usually associated with generalized lymphadenopathy
b. is associated with gross splenomegaly
c. is usually associated with marked prostration and delirium
d. infection is contracted from tsetse flies
e. is associated with hypergammaglobulinaemia

177. **Falciparum malaria**
a. acute infection is not associated with splenomegaly
b. is associated with periodic fever in a minority of cases
c. has an incubation period of 8–15 days
d. may present as a gastroenteritis
e. may be treated with primaquine

178. **The main biologically active form of vitamin D**
a. is 24,25-dihydroxyvitamin D
b. is produced by hydroxylation in the kidney
c. production is increased by parathyroid hormone
d. promotes intestinal phosphate absorption
e. decreases renal tubular calcium resorption

179. **Vitamin K**
a. is a fat-soluble vitamin
b. is essential for coagulation factor V synthesis
c. becomes deficient in prolonged obstructive jaundice
d. is produced by bacteria within the bowel
e. crosses the placenta

180. **Primary Sjögren's syndrome**
a. is more commonly associated with the presence of anti-SS-B (anti-Ro) antibodies than is the case where associated with rheumatoid arthritis
b. is associated with renal dysfunction, of which proteinuria is the earliest feature

40

c. is characterized by hypergammaglobulinaemia
d. is not associated with rheumatoid factor
e. is associated with an increased incidence of lymphoid neoplasia

181. **Causes of bilateral lower motor neuron facial nerve lesions include**
a. Brown-Séquard syndrome
b. acute postinfective polyneuritis
c. sarcoidosis
d. lepromatous leprosy
e. poliomyelitis

182. **Insulin**
a. stimulates glucokinase activity
b. regulates hepatic glucose metabolism by alteration of glucose transport into cells
c. activates glycogen synthetase
d. deficiency is associated with reduced hepatic free fatty acid synthesis
e. deficiency is associated with increased triglyceride breakdown in adipose tissue

183. **Recognized complications of ulcerative colitis include**
a. benign stricture of the colon
b. erythema nodosum
c. monoarticular acute arthritis of the knee
d. cirrhosis
e. iritis

184. **Juvenile rheumatoid arthritis**
a. is most commonly associated with uveitis in boys presenting with systemic disease
b. is almost always associated with a positive test for rheumatoid factor
c. is unlikely to be complicated by uveitis in the absence of clinical symptoms
d. with an oligoarticular presentation is usually antinuclear antibody-positive
e. with a polyarticular involvement is complicated by ankylosis

of the posterior apophyseal joints of the upper cervical spine

185. **Primary hyperparathyroidism**
   a. is almost always associated with generalized muscle weakness
   b. is a cause of recurrent renal calculi
   c. is associated with corneal calcium deposition
   d. is a cause of periosteal new bone formation
   e. is associated with pyrophosphate arthropathy (pseudogout)

186. **With respect to Cushing's syndrome**
   a. dexamethasone (2 mg 6-hourly for 3 days) usually suppresses corticosteroid production in Cushing's disease (pituitary adenoma)
   b. lack of suppression by dexamethasone (7 mg 6-hourly for 3 days) in cases of ectopic ACTH production would be expected
   c. 17-hydroxysteroid excretion is unaffected by coexisting hepatic disease and is therefore the test of choice in this situation
   d. urinary 17-ketosteroid excretion more accurately reflects glucocorticoid excess than does 17-hydroxysteroid excretion
   e. measurement of urinary free cortisol is probably the best screening test for Cushing's syndrome

187. **Which of the following statements are true with respect to hypothyroidism?**
   a. thyroxine (T_4) production is about 25% of normal, or less, in patients with overt hypothyroidism
   b. T_4 is proportionally more reduced than is triiodothyronine (T_3)
   c. the proportion of T_3 secreted by the thyroid gland is greater than normal
   d. most patients who are ill, but do not have thyroid disease, have low T_3 levels
   e. 98% of cases are primary

188. **The ulnar nerve**
   a. innervates the first dorsal interosseus muscle

b. originates from the medial cord of the brachial plexus
c. has no branches above the elbow
d. innervates the medial half of the flexor digitorum profundus
e. innervates the adductor pollicis muscle

189. α_1-Antitrypsin
a. is secreted by type 1 pneumocytes
b. inhibits neutrophil elastase activity
c. levels are not decreased in heterozygotes (Pi MZ)
d. deficiency is associated with predominantly apical pulmonary emphysema
e. deficiency is associated with significantly more pulmonary disease in those who smoke

190. Phenytoin
a. is rapidly absorbed from the gastrointestinal tract
b. therapy is associated with osteomalacia
c. is significantly bound to plasma albumin
d. levels are increased by concurrent carbamazepine therapy
e. levels are increased by concurrent dicoumarol therapy

191. Tardive dyskinesia
a. is characterized by immobility
b. usually responds rapidly to anticholinergic therapy
c. usually develops within 3 months of initiation of phenothiazine therapy
d. usually resolves within 3 months of the withdrawal of phenothiazine therapy
e. is recognized to respond to anticholinergic treatment

192. With which of the following is concurrent administration of warfarin liable to result in dangerous potentiation of the PT?
a. clofibrate
b. spironolactone
c. phenobarbitone
d. ascorbic acid
e. cholestyramine

193. As regards *Helicobacter pylori*
a. it is unlikely to be identified in the gastric mucosa of patients

43

with duodenal ulceration and marked diffuse antral gastritis
b. infection is less common in those aged over 65 years compared with the 40–60-year-old group
c. <50% of patients with duodenal ulceration have *H. pylori* identified in their antral mucosa
d. gastrin release is enhanced in patients with *H. pylori* infection
e. sustained eradication of *H. pylori* occurs in <20% of those treated with bismuth plus metronidazole

194. Hereditary angio-oedema
a. is associated with C4 deficiency
b. is associated with an increased risk of SLE
c. is often associated with an urticarial rash which itches
d. is characterized by attacks of angio-oedema which usually resolve within 4 h
e. is prevented by oestrogen therapy

195. Which of the following occur in Crohn's disease of the colon, but not in ulcerative colitis?
a. radiological abnormality of the ileum
b. crypt abscesses
c. radiological narrowing of the bowel
d. radiological sparing of the rectum
e. fibrosis of the bowel wall

196. An elevated ESR is found in association with
a. hypoalbuminaemia
b. cold agglutinins
c. anaemia
d. pregnancy
e. hypofibrinogenaemia

197. IgA nephropathy
a. carries a poor prognosis for renal function if nephrotic syndrome is associated
b. is the commonest form of glomerulonephritis to be associated with macroscopic haematuria
c. is almost always associated with persistent proteinuria

44

    d. progresses to chronic renal failure in <35% of cases

    e. is associated with increased circulating IgA levels

198. The oesophagus

    a. is lined by stratified columnar epithelium

    b. is surrounded by serosa

    c. middle third venous drainage is to the azygous system

    d. contains no Auerbach's plexus

    e. passes through the diaphragm through the same hiatus as does the inferior vena cava

199. The duodenum

    a. is the site of maximal iron absorption

    b. is crossed anteriorly by the superior mesenteric artery

    c. is intraperitoneal for its first 5 cm

    d. terminates at the ligament of Treitz

    e. contains Brunner's glands

200. In a patient with steatorrhoea, which of the following findings favour a diagnosis of coeliac disease rather than chronic pancreatic insufficiency?

    a. a faecal fat excretion of 40 g/day

    b. normal intestinal xylose absorption

    c. hypoalbuminaemia

    d. a bleeding diathesis

    e. a megaloblastic anaemia due to folate deficiency

201. Bilirubin

    a. in unconjugated form is predominantly bound to albumin

    b. in conjugated form is bound more strongly to albumin than in unconjugated form

    c. is excreted predominantly conjugated with glucuronic acid

    d. in conjugated form is about 25% reabsorbed from the small bowel

    e. in unconjugated form is excreted in the urine when blood levels reach about twice the normal level

202. Delayed gastric emptying is associated with

    a. cholecystokinin infusion

    b. truncal vagotomy

c. VIP infusion
d. diabetic ketoacidosis
e. diabetic neuropathy

203. **Typical characteristics of Argyll Robertson pupils complicating neurosyphilis include**
a. small size
b. normal dilatation after atropine instillation
c. depigmentation of the iris
d. dilatation on convergence
e. preservation of the ciliospinal reflex

204. **The spinal cord**
a. terminates at the level of the lower border of the third lumbar vertebra
b. has an average length of 20 cm
c. is suspended laterally by the ligamentum flavum
d. is supplied with blood from the vertebral arteries by way of the anterior spinal arteries
e. is supplied with blood from radicular arteries which reach the cord via the intervertebral foramina

205. **Chlorpromazine therapy for 1 year is associated with**
a. an increased plasma cholesterol level
b. a decreased plasma prolactin level
c. increased urine homovanillic acid excretion
d. an increased convulsion threshold in epileptics
e. potentiation of the hypotensive action of guanethidine

206. **α-Methyldopa**
a. inhibits decarboxylation of dopa
b. therapy is associated with reduced plasma renin levels
c. reduces renal blood flow
d. therapy is associated with raised serum prolactin levels
e. does not result in a fall of blood pressure until >60 min have elapsed after intravenous administration

207. **Sideroblastic anaemia**
a. may be familial
b. is a feature of lead poisoning

c. is characterized by ring sideroblasts in the bone marrow
d. may complicate treatment of tuberculosis
e. is never of such severity as to require blood transfusion

208. **Karsakoff's syndrome is characteristically associated with**
a. disorientation
b. auditory hallucinations
c. confabulation
d. glial proliferation in the mamillary bodies
e. severe defect of both long- and short-term memory

209. **Infection with the *Mycobacterium avium* complex (MAC)**
a. generally follows contact with diseased birds
b. is diagnosed by culture of the organism from the sputum
c. characteristically causes cavities which are smaller and thinner-walled than those associated with *M. tuberculosis* infection.
d. is a common cause of hepatosplenomegaly with raised alkaline phosphatase in patients with AIDS
e. is generally sensitive to clarithromycin

210. **In muscular dystrophy of the Duchenne type**
a. there is almost always a family history of the condition
b. electrocardiographic abnormality develops in almost all cases
c. tendon reflexes are typically preserved until the advanced stages of disease
d. creatine kinase (CK) estimation on heelprick samples from newborn males is an effective method of early diagnosis
e. the calf muscles are usually the site of the earliest detectable weakness

211. **Which of the following statements are true?**
a. the sinoatrial node is always supplied by a branch of the right coronary artery
b. the atrioventricular node is usually supplied by a branch of the left coronary artery
c. the posterior interventricular septum may be supplied by branches of the left coronary artery

d. the posterior descending coronary artery is usually a branch of the right coronary artery

e. the anterior fascicle of the left bundle branch is usually supplied by the anterior descending branch of the left coronary artery

212. **In Wenckebach (type I) second-degree heart block**
a. the block is usually at the level of the atrioventricular node
b. on the ECG the shortest RR interval typically occurs just before the dropped beat
c. the ventricular rate typically increases with exercise
d. progression to complete heart block may occur
e. on the ECG the duration of the QRS complex is frequently increased

213. **A 21-year-old woman develops rigors, a maculopapular rash and a painful swollen right knee and left wrist. Her boyfriend has recently been treated for gonorrhoea; a diagnosis of disseminated gonococcal infection is made. Which of the following statements are correct?**
a. she is very likely to have a positive blood culture
b. the arthritis is an immune phenomenon and the synovial fluid will grow gonococci in <30% of cases of disseminated gonococcal infection
c. disseminated gonococcal infection very rarely occurs in the absence of associated genitourinary symptoms
d. it is unusual for more than one or two joints to be involved in disseminated gonococcal infection
e. disseminated gonococcal infection is a recognized cause of tenosynovitis

214. **Which of the following features favour a diagnosis of limb-girdle muscular dystrophy rather than facioscapulohumeral muscular dystrophy?**
a. a dominant pattern of inheritance
b. premature death due to disease progression
c. early tibialis anterior weakness
d. severe scoliosis
e. the identification of abortive cases within the family

215. **Isolation of *Clostridium difficile* from the stool sample**
   a. is more common in neonates than in adults
   b. is almost always associated with antibiotic-associated colitis (AAC)
   c. does not necessarily imply toxin production
   d. will be associated with invasion of the colonic mucosa by *C. difficile* in the presence of AAC
   e. is less common than the isolation of *Staphylococcus aureus* in cases of established AAC

216. **Farmers' lung**
   a. results from inhalation of spores of *A. fumigatus* to which the subject has become sensitized
   b. is more prevalent in those farming in regions with lower rainfall
   c. is almost invariable in those with positive precipitating antibodies to the appropriate antigen
   d. is less likely in farmers who smoke
   e. can be avoided by a change to silage feeding

217. **In pulmonary embolism**
   a. when a ventilation/perfusion ($\dot{V}/\dot{Q}$) scan is reported as 'low-risk' a pulmonary angiogram reveals pulmonary embolism in <10% of cases
   b. >90% of patients with positive lung scans will be found to have positive venograms
   c. Heparin enhances clot lysis by augmenting the action of antithrombin III
   d. patients with pulmonary embolism show more heparin resistance than do those without embolism
   e. with thrombolytic treatment resolution of clot is more rapid than when heparin is used alone

218. **In medullary carcinoma of the thyroid**
   a. basal calcitonin levels are often elevated
   b. hypocalcaemia is typical
   c. calcitonin levels may be increased by calcium infusion
   d. diarrhoea is a recognized clinical manifestation
   e. metastases can usually be identified by radioactive iodine uptake

49

219. **Which of the following statements are correct?**
   a. the external branch of the superior laryngeal nerve innervates the cricothyroid muscle
   b. the recurrent laryngeal nerve innervates the cricopharyngeus muscle
   c. the superior laryngeal nerve is a branch of the vagus
   d. bilateral recurrent laryngeal nerve lesions are invariably associated with aphonia
   e. the cricothyroid muscle is the major abductor of the vocal cords

220. **Thrombosis of the hepatic veins**
   a. results in the development of a characteristic periportal hepatic necrosis on liver histology
   b. results in the development of ascites, typically with the characteristics of a transudate
   c. is usually associated with predominant necrosis of the caudate lobe
   d. causes histological changes in the liver indistinguishable from those resulting from right heart failure
   e. results in the development of hepatomegaly

221. **In a patient with progressive radiological pulmonary infiltration due to *Pneumocystis carinii***
   a. a titre of >1/16 to *P. carinii* is diagnostic
   b. auscultatory signs would be expected to be worse than anticipated from the chest X-ray appearance
   c. the diagnosis cannot be expected to be made in >30% of cases on sputum examination
   d. haemoptysis is a common feature
   e. pulmonary fibrosis occurs in most cases following treatment

222. **Which of the following statements are correct?**
   a. reduced haemoglobin buffers hydrogen ion more effectively than oxyhaemoglobin
   b. the 'chloride shift' refers to a movement of chloride ions into the red cell
   c. most carbon dioxide in venous blood is transported bound to albumin

50

d. carbon dioxide binds with reduced haemoglobin

e. the enzyme carbonic anhydrase is present in red cells

223. Which of the following statements are correct?

a. granulocyte-colony stimulating factor (G-CSF) is a polypeptide

b. neutrophil precursor cell division is enhanced by G-CSF but the rate of maturation is not accelerated

c. peak circulating neutrophil count occurs 36–48 h after subcutaneous G-CSF administration

d. circulating precursor cells are explained by recent GM-CSF treatment

e. following bone marrow transplantation more rapid restoration of neutrophil numbers is seen in GM-CSF-treated patients

224. The oxygen affinity of haemoglobin

a. is reduced if the P_{CO_2} is increased

b. of the fetal type (HbF) is higher than normal adult haemoglobin

c. is increased by raised red-cell 2,3 DPG concentration

d. is decreased in the presence of acidosis

e. is increased if the temperature is raised by $3\,^\circ C$

225. In Down's syndrome (trisomy 21) there is

a. increased maternal α-fetoprotein levels

b. male infertility

c. an increased incidence of leukaemoid reactions but no true increased risk of leukaemia

d. stong association with paternal age independent of the known increased risk with increasing maternal age

e. neurochemical change characteristic of Alzheimer's disease in the brains of all individuals aged over 40 years

226. Which of the following statements are true?

a. the normal haemoglobin concentration of a 3-month-old child is lower than that of an adult

b. reticulocytes are smaller than mature red blood cells

c. reticulocytes tend to persist in the circulation for a longer period when erythropoiesis is very active

d. the MCH is generally low in megaloblastic anaemias

51

e. the MCH concentration (MCHC) is generally normal in megaloblastic anaemia

227. In the proximal tubule of the nephron
- **a.** the tubular fluid remains essentially iso-osmotic
- **b.** glucose is reabsorbed
- **c.** sodium reabsorption is passive
- **d.** permeability to water is increased by antidiuretic hormone (ADH)
- **e.** a varying proportion of the filtrate is reabsorbed at different rates of glomerular filtration

228. Lesions inside the mouth characteristically occur in
- **a.** pemphigus vulgaris
- **b.** pityriasis rosea
- **c.** lichen planus
- **d.** psoriasis
- **e.** dermatitis herpetiformis

229. During an asthmatic attack typical findings include
- **a.** hypoxia
- **b.** a reduced total lung capacity
- **c.** a reduced inspiratory capacity
- **d.** reduced static compliance
- **e.** an increased functional residual capacity

230. Sexual precocity
- **a.** is a cause of short stature
- **b.** is a recognized result of high circulating T_4 levels
- **c.** is associated with ovulation when an oestrogen-secreting ovarian tumour is the cause
- **d.** occurs in girls with congenital adrenal hyperplasia due to 21β-hydroxylase deficiency
- **e.** is most commonly caused by a hypothalamic tumour

231. With regard to prognosis in acute leukaemia
- **a.** in acute myeloid leukaemia (AML) $t(8;21)$ or $inv(16)$ karyotype is associated with a good chance of complete remission

b. patients with AML who have an additional chromosome 8 on cytogenetic examination have a low remission rate and a poor chance of attaining long-term remission

c. patients who have a preceding myelodysplastic syndrome have a better chance of remission from AML than those who develop AML without any preceding myelodysplasia

d. patients with B-cell acute lymphoblastic leukaemia (ALL) have a lower complete remission rate than those with T-cell ALL

e. patients with ALL who have diploid (normal karyotype) cells have a better remission rate than those with cytogenetic abnormality

232. Bacteria in the bowel
a. are always an abnormal finding in the upper ileum
b. cause bile salt conjugation
c. metabolize tryptophan to indican
d. decompose urea
e. are liable to be associated with vitamin B_{12} deficiency if they are present in excessive numbers

233. Which of the following are consistent with a diagnosis of Wilson's disease?
a. high biliary copper excretion
b. high caeruloplasmin levels during infection
c. high serum copper level in fulminant hepatic failure
d. low serum copper level
e. resolution of dystonia within 7 days of initiation of high-dose penicillamine treatment

234. Acetylcholine
a. is the neurotransmitter substance at sympathetic ganglia
b. action at the synapse is predominantly limited by reuptake into nerve endings
c. metabolism is catalysed by catechol O-methyltransferase
d. is the neurotransmitter at postganglionic sympathetic endings which stimulate sweating
e. release from sympathetic nerve fibres in the adrenal medulla stimulates adrenaline release

235. **Which of the following typically stimulate the release of ADH?**
    a. alcohol
    b. intravenous infusion of 500 ml plasma
    c. hypertension
    d. morphine administration
    e. pain

236. *Toxoplasma gondii*
    a. is a helminth
    b. is transmitted to humans by ingestion of tissue cysts in raw or undercooked meat
    c. is the major cause of multifocal necrotizing encephalitis in patients with AIDS
    d. congenital infection is reduced by maternal treatment during pregnancy
    e. is effectively treated by trimethoprim–sulphamethoxazole (high-dose)

237. **Which of the following directly stimulate gastric secretion of gastrin and result in increased gastric acidity?**
    a. a 20% glucose infusion into the gastric antrum
    b. distension of the gastric antrum following atropine treatment
    c. antacid ingestion
    d. amino acid infusion into the gastric antrum
    e. vagal stimulation

238. **B lymphocytes**
    a. are normally the predominant type of circulating lymphocyte
    b. proliferate in response to IL-2
    c. are associated with the development of humoral immunity
    d. are the predominant cell type in the paracortical region of the lymph nodes
    e. are characterized by rosette formation when mixed with sheep red cells

239. **Which of the following statements about the serological tests for syphilis are correct?**
    a. the Venereal Disease Research Laboratory (VDRL; reagin) test becomes negative within 2 months of effective antibiotic treatment of primary syphilis

b. the VDRL (reagin) test gives a false-positive result in >5% of patients over 70 years of age
c. the antigen used in the reagin tests is a treponemal extract
d. leptospirosis is a recognized cause of a false-positive *Treponema pallidum* haemagglutination (TPHA) test
e. a continuing positive TPHA test is indicative of inadequately treated secondary syphilis

240. *H. influenzae*
a. is a Gram-positive bacterium
b. is not found in the nasopharynx of healthy individuals
c. produces spores
d. is identified by Optochin sensitivity
e. of the strain associated with most cases of meningitis has no capsule

241. **With regard to antiglomerular basement membrane antibody-mediated nephritis (Goodpasture's syndrome)**
a. pulmonary disease is unlikely in the absence of haemoptysis
b. that which has caused oliguric renal failure is still likely to respond to plasmapheresis
c. is unlikely to relapse when antiglomerular basement membrane antibodies are normalized
d. glomerular crescents on renal biopsy are incompatible with the diagnosis
e. it is more likely to be associated with pulmonary haemorrhage in a patient who smokes

242. **In classical anterior internuclear ophthalmoplegia complicating multiple sclerosis there is**
a. an inability to converge the eyes
b. usually a weakness of movement of the abducting eye on lateral gaze
c. nystagmus of the adducting eye on lateral gaze
d. a lesion in the medial lemniscus which results in the defect
e. ataxic nystagmus

243. **Typical features of HOCM include**
a. increased obstruction to ventricular emptying after amyl nitrate inhalation

b. a Mendelian recessive mode of inheritance
c. a slow rising carotid pulse
d. a low end-diastolic ventricular pressure
e. mitral regurgitation

244. Deficiency of clotting factor VII
a. is associated with a prolongation of the PT
b. is associated with a prolongation of the partial
thromboplastin time
c. is associated with a prolonged thrombin time
d. is associated with a prolonged bleeding time
e. is associated with a positive tourniquet (Hess) test

245. Extrinsic allergic alveolitis
a. is typically associated with the development of wheeze on
re-exposure to the antigen
b. causes symptoms which generally resolve within 1 h of
cessation of exposure to the antigen
c. leads to a restrictive defect of lung function
d. is almost invariably associated with an eosinophilia in the
peripheral blood
e. almost invariably occurs in atopic individuals

246. Features of haemochromatosis include
a. early hepatocellular failure
b. associated chondrocalcinosis
c. a family history in almost all cases
d. an increased risk of developing hepatocellular carcinoma
e. almost invariable occurence in atopic individuals

**247. Which of the following statements about sarcoidosis are
correct?**
a. there is usually a hypergammaglobulinaemia
b. angiotensin-converting enzyme (ACE) levels are increased in
<30% of cases of acute sarcoidosis
c. there is an impaired delayed hypersensitivity reaction to
intradermal *Candida albicans*
d. clubbing of the fingers is usual when parenchymal lung
disease is present
e. when parenchymal lung disease develops there is impaired

gas transfer before a reduction of the vital capacity can be detected

248. Typical findings on investigation of a neuropathy associated with segmental demyelination include

a. polyphasic action potentials on electromyography
b. marked fibrillation potentials on electromyography
c. fasciculation
d. marked reduction of the nerve conduction velocity
e. a reduced amplitude of the action potential produced by nerve stimulation

249. Juxtaductal aortic coarctation

a. usually occurs just above the origin of the left subclavian artery
b. is not associated with rib notching in infants
c. is a recognized site of bacterial infection
d. is associated with bicuspid aortic value
e. is associated with pulmonary valve stenosis

250. Effects of bilateral diaphragmatic paralysis include

a. a reduced vital capacity
b. decreased maximal expiratory force
c. dyspnoea which is exacerbated by lying down
d. hypoxia which is exacerbated by lying down
e. increased respiratory difficulty when immersed in water

251. Angiotensin converting enzyme inhibitor therapy results in

a. reduced plasma renin levels
b. raised bradykinin levels
c. increased catecholamine levels
d. improved cardiac output in congestive cardiac failure irrespective of pretreatment renin levels
e. less arterial desaturation than is associated with treatment with sodium nitroprusside

252. *Torsade de pointes*

a. is a complication of procainamide treatment
b. is associated with a prolonged QT interval
c. is a recognized complication of hypokalaemia

57

d. is likely to respond to quinidine

e. is a recognized cause of syncope in complete heart block

253. Somatostatin

a. stimulates pancreatic glucagon release

b. reduces stimulated gastric acid secretion

c. enhances gastric emptying

d. enhances cholecystokinin-induced gallbladder contraction

e. increases pancreatic exocrine enzyme secretion

254. Concerning infective diarrhoea and antimicrobial drugs

a. ampicillin is indicated in cases of enteritis due to non-typhoidal salmonella since treatment reduces the duration of intestinal carriage of the organism

b. *Shigella flexneri* is almost always sensitive to ampicillin

c. in colitis due to *Campylobacter jejuni* faecal excretion of the organism is reduced by erythromycin treatment

d. severe diarrhoea due to *C. jejuni* is usually ameliorated by ampicillin

e. travellers' diarrhoea is reduced in duration and severity by treatment with trimethoprim-sulphamethoxazole

255. With which of the following is infection associated with leucocytes and red cells on faecal microscopy?

a. *Giardia lamblia*

b. *C. jejuni*

c. *Vibrio cholerae*

d. rotavirus

e. enteropathogenic *Escherichia coli* (EPEC)

256. As regards hepatitis B serology

a. demonstration of DNA polymerase activity is an expected observation in a patient with HBeAg

b. HBcAg is present in high titre during acute icteric HBV hepatitis

c. HBeAg is detected in a significant number of patients with negative tests for HBsAg

d. the absence of HBsAg positivity at the time of the onset of hepatitis excludes HBV as the cause

e. fewer than 2% of chronic carriers cease to be HBeAg-positive each year that they are followed

257. *Coxiella burnetii* (the aetiological agent of Q fever)
a. does not infect domestic animals (cats and dogs)
b. is a cause of hepatitis
c. is associated with a positive Weil–Felix reaction
d. is very sensitive to erythromycin
e. is an occupational risk in abattoir workers

258. Protein C
a. levels are increased by warfarin therapy
b. deficiency is associated with an a haemorrhagic diathesis
c. deficiency is associated with a prolongation of the PT
d. acts predominantly by inhibiting thrombin action
e. deficiency is inherited as a sex-linked recessive

259. Antithrombin III deficiency syndrome
a. is inherited as an autosomal dominant
b. is associated with increased sensitivity to heparin
c. is ameliorated by oral contraceptives since these result in increased antithrombin III levels
d. can be treated acutely by infusion of fresh frozen plasma
e. treated with oral anticoagulant is associated with increased antithrombin III levels

260. *Entamoeba histolytica*
a. excysts in the stomach and trophozoites then penetrate into the portal blood
b. infection results from ingestion of trophozoites in contaminated water
c. is very unlikely to be the cause of a liver abscess in a patient who has returned from an endemic area more than 2 weeks previously
d. infection of the colon is more likely to result in high numbers of faecal leucocytes than where *Shigella* is the cause
e. is a well-recognized cause of colonic perforation

Part 2
Answers and Notes

1. Cystinuria
ANSWER: a

NOTES
• Cystinuria is an autosomal recessive disorder characterized by a specific dibasic aminoaciduria, the result of a defective tubular reabsorption mechanism.
• Cystine, lysine, arginine and ornithine are excreted in great excess in the urine of homozygotes.
• The clinical features result from the insolubility of cystine in the urinary tract with calculus formation. Hexagonal cystine crystals are present in the urine.
• Calculi are radiopaque due to their sulphur content. About 10% of calculi which are produced by patients with cystinuria contain no cystine; most others contain a variable proportion of calcium phosphate.
• The cyanide–nitroprusside urine test is positive in cystinuria and in homocystinuria.
• Treatment of cystinuria includes high fluid intake (throughout the 24-h period to reduce cystine precipitation). Urinary alkalization (cystine is more soluble in alkaline urine) is probably not particularly effective since solubility of cystine only increases significantly at pH >7.5. D-penicillamine binds with cystine, increasing solubility.
• Lysine is the only essential dibasic amino acid and diet usually contains enough to compensate for the urinary loss.
• Ammonium chloride results in an acid load and urinary acidification; this is detrimental in cystinuria.
• Cystinosis is a different disease where there is intracellular cystine accumulation in many tissues. Cystine urinary calculi are not a feature; deposition of cystine in the renal tubular cells results in a generalized aminoaciduria.
• Homocystinuria is characterized by ectopia lentis, arachnodactyly

and other features similar to those seen in Marfan's syndrome; calculi are not associated.

SCRIVER *et al.* (1989) pp. 698, 2479, 2619

2. Ketones
ANSWERS: a c d e

NOTES
• In the fed state insulin levels are high and intracellular malonyl–coenzyme A (CoA) levels increase. Malonyl–CoA is a key intermediate, high levels of which inhibit carnitine palmitoyltransferase I (CPT-1), thus favouring triglyceride synthesis and retarding fatty acid oxidation and ketone body formation.
• CPT-1 transesterifies fatty acetyl CoA to fatty acyl carnitine, thus enabling it to enter mitochondria, the site of fatty acid oxidation to ketones.
• Glucagon has powerful ketogenic and antilipogenic actions.
• Long-chain fatty acids from triglyceride stores in adipose tissue are the principal substrate for ketone production in the liver (in disease states fatty infiltration of the liver with triglyceride is an alternative source).
• The major ketone bodies are acetoacetate and β-hydroxybutyrate.
• With the exception of the liver, most organs can oxidize ketone bodies. Rates of utilization appears to be regulated primarily by tissue concentration.
• In diabetic ketoacidosis the β-hydroxybutyrate concentration is at least twice that of acetoacetate. The ratio depends on the redox state of the hepatocytes, and higher amounts of β-hydroxybutyrate with less acetoacetate is seen in shocked patients with liver hypoxia or in patients with ethanol ingestion. Ketone test strips react with acetoacetate and may occasionally give a false-negative result in these situations.

DEGROOT (1995) pp. 1345, 1407, 1509, 1512

3. Corticospinal tract
ANSWERS: a b d

NOTES
• The corticospinal tracts are the most important motor tracts. They

mediate initiation and control of voluntary muscular movement.

• The fibres originate from the cells of cerebral cortex, predominantly from the precentral motor region.

• The fibres run in the corona radiata from the cortex to the internal capsule. In the internal capsule the corticospinal tract occupies the posterior third of the anterior limb and the anterior two-thirds of the posterior limb.

• The head of the caudate nucleus and the optic thalamus lie medial to the internal capsule; the lentiform nucleus is lateral.

• Below the internal capsule the corticospinal tracts run in the cerebral peduncles on the anterior aspect of the midbrain. The substantia nigra is the immediate posterior relation. Here the close relation to the third-nerve nucleus may result in lesions occurring to both (Weber's syndrome, third-nerve lesion and contralateral hemiplegia).

• At the pons the transversely running fibres break the tracts into scattered bundles, which rejoin caudally to run in the pyramids on the anterior aspect of the medulla. Lesions to the corticospinal tract in the pons result in a contralateral hemiplegia but the higher cranial nerves (controlling eye movement) are preserved. The facial nerve nucleus may also be involved, resulting in facial paralysis on the opposite side to the hemiplegia.

• In the medulla most of the fibres decussate, thereafter running in the lateral funiculus of the spinal cord. A small proportion of the fibres remain uncrossed and descend in the anterior white matter. These uncrossed fibres decussate at the segmental level of the cord at which they terminate.

• The thalamocortical tract runs in the posterior limb of the internal capsule; this relays sensory information to the postcentral and other cortical sensory areas. The visual fibres in the geniculocalcarine pathway run in the posterior limb of the internal capsule.

WALTON (1993) p. 18

4. Acute tubular necrosis
ANSWERS: b c d e

NOTES

• In acute tubular necrosis the urinary sodium is classically greater than 40 mmol/l. The urine osmolality is <350 mosmol/kg.

• The renal failure index (RFI) is the urinary sodium (per litre) (UNa) divided by the urine/plasma (U/P) creatinine ratio. RFI values >1 favour acute tubular necrosis.

• The FE_{Na} is about 90% sensitive and specific in differentiating prerenal failure from acute tubular necrosis. Values of >1% suggest acute tubular necrosis.

• Brownish pigmented casts with numerous renal tubular epithelial cells are seen in >75% of cases of acute tubular necrosis. Red-cell casts are not associated and suggest glomerulonephritis.

• Some unselective proteinuria is usual, but heavy proteinuria (>2 g/day) suggests glomerular disease.

SCHRIER & GOTTSCHALK (1993) p. 1287

5. *Salmonella typhi*
ANSWER: all incorrect

NOTES
• *S. typhi* is a non-spore-forming Gram-negative rod.

• The only known reservoir of *S. typhi* is humans, so direct or indirect contact with a patient with typhoid fever or a chronic carrier is necessary for infection. Transmission of *S. typhi* is faecal–oral.

• Most outbreaks are due to water contamination by faeces but faecal contamination of the hands of carriers who are employed in food preparation is also a risk. Shellfish filter water and concentrate organisms if they are present. Milk and cream are good media for *S. typhi* multiplication.

• Incubation period is usually 10–14 days.

• Blood culture is positive in 80% of patients (who have had no antibiotic) during the first week of illness. Bone marrow culture is more sensitive. Faecal culture is positive during the second and third weeks. Culture of rose spots may also reveal organisms.

• Serology is unreliable. Antibody to O antigen (Widal test) shows a fourfold rise in <50% of untreated cases and even less when antibiotics are given.

• Complications include relapse (in about 10% of cases; this may be increased by chloramphenicol treatment), gastrointestinal haemorrhage and perforation.

• Chloramphenicol, ampicillin and co-trimoxazole reduce the duration of the disease.

• Those excreting for >1 year are termed chronic carriers. The chronic carrier rate is 1–3%. The Vi antibody is present in about 70% of carriers (at 1 : 5 dilution), but in only 1% of the normal population.
• Faecal excretion is much more common in carriers than is urinary excretion. Carriers are much more commonly female and risk increases with age. Gallbladder disease appears an important factor favouring carriage.
• Ampicillin appears to be more effective than chloramphenicol in terminating the carrier state. If the gallbladder is diseased, as is usually the case, removal with concurrent ampicillin treatment results in a cure of the carrier state in >75% of cases.

MANDELL, BENNETT & DOLIN (1995) p. 1700

6. Ptosis
ANSWERS: a b c d

NOTES
• The third nerve (oculomotor) supplies all the external ocular muscles, with the exception of the lateral rectus and superior oblique muscles. In addition it carries parasympathetic fibres.
• A complete third-nerve lesion results in ptosis (due to loss of parasympathetic supply of the levator palpebrae superioris), mydriasis, paralysis of accommodation and deviation of the eye laterally and downward (due to unopposed superior oblique and lateral rectus activity).
• Damage to the cervical sympathetic nervous system results in slight ptosis, reduced size of the pupil on the same side (miosis) and retraction of the eye (enophthalmos).
• Ptosis of congenital origin may be either unilateral or bilateral.

HART (1985) p. 691
WALTON (1993) p. 98

7. Systemic lupus erythematosus
ANSWER: all incorrect

NOTES
• Antinuclear factor (ANF), often in high titre, is almost always present in SLE (severe uraemia may render the result negative). ANF

is associated with many other conditions (usually of lower titre than found in SLE), including systemic sclerosis, rheumatoid arthritis, chronic active hepatitis, Sjögren's syndrome, Still's disease, fibrosing alveolitis and drug reactions.

• Antibodies to double-stranded (native) DNA are the single most specific marker of SLE; binding of antibody (DNA-binding) tends to correlate with disease activity.

• Low C1, C3, C4 (classic pathway) complement levels are indicative of renal involvement in SLE. C2 levels (alternative pathway) are less often depressed.

• Cryoglobulins occur; they are also generally correlated with disease activity.

• A positive Coombs test is common but haemolytic anaemia occurs in less then 15% of cases. Antiplatelet antibodies are commonly present. Lymphocytotoxic antibodies are present in the serum of most (>80%) patients with SLE.

• Circulating anticoagulant occurs in >20%. It rarely causes marked bleeding tendency *in vivo* but is associated with prolongation of the partial thromboplastin time (PTT). There is an associated predisposition to venous and arterial thrombosis.

• Skin biopsy shows gammaglobulin and complement in 90% of cases, characteristically in a band of granular deposits at the dermoepidermal junction.

• Defects of suppressor T-cell function are constant findings in active SLE.

KELLEY *et al.* (1993) p. 1017

8. Glycosylated haemoglobin
ANSWERS: b c e

NOTES

• Glycosylated haemoglobin (HbA_{1c}), the most abundant minor haemoglobin in human erythrocytes, is increased in diabetics.

• In HbA_{1c} a hexose sugar is attached to the N-terminal valines of the normal β chains of HbA_1.

• The rate of formation of HbA_{1c} is directly proportional to the time–average concentration of glucose within the erythrocyte.

• When poorly controlled diabetes is carefully controlled then HbA_{1c} levels fall after a lag of 5–6 weeks.

• Diabetic women becoming pregnant who are found to have high HbA$_{1c}$ levels appear to be at increased risk of having babies with congential abnormality. Very high levels are associated with higher risk.

DEGROOT *et al.* (1995) p. 1421

9. Midbrain anatomy
ANSWERS: a d e

NOTES
• The midbrain is traversed by the aqueduct which joins the third and fourth ventricles.
• The oculomotor (III) and Edinger–Westphal nuclei lie in the periaqueductal grey matter at the level of the superior colliculus. The trochlear (IV) nucleus is similarly situated at the level of the inferior colliculus.
• The third nerve emerges from the ventral aspect of the midbrain in the space between the cerebral peduncles. The fourth nerve emerges dorsally from the upper end of the superior medullary velum (which forms the roof of the fourth ventricle).
• The substantia nigra lies in a position immediately dorsal to the cerebral peduncles in the midbrain.
• The red nucleus is situated in the midbrain at the level of the superior colliculus.
• The facial nucleus is situated in the pons.
• The nucleus ambiguus is the common motor nucleus of the glossopharyngeal (IX), vagus (X) and accessory (XI) nerves. It is situated in the medulla.

WALTON (1993) p. 24

10. Cyclosporin actions
ANSWER: all incorrect

NOTES
• Cyclosporin blocks cytotoxic T-cell activation by a number of different effects.
• IL-2 production by activated helper T cells is profoundly inhibited by cyclosporin. At higher doses IL-2 receptor expression is reduced.

Athough cyclosporin inhibits activation of helper T cells, it does not affect their clonal expansion in response to IL-2.
• Suppressor T-cell activity occurs at concentrations of cyclosporin which inhibit the induction of cytotoxic T cells.
• Reticulophagocytic function and myeloid synthesis are not affected by cyclosporin.
• Increased prolactin secretion in patients on cyclosporin is well-documented.
• Cyclosporin binds to cyclophillins which are abundant in lymphoid tissue.
• 60–70% of cyclosporin in whole blood is contained in red cells. Up to 20% is contained in lymphocytes (disproportionately high in respect to their small representation in whole blood).
• Nephrotoxicity occurs in up to 75% of treated patients.

GILMAN *et al.* (1990) p. 1267

11. von Willebrand's disease (vWD)
ANSWERS: b d e

NOTES
• Inheritance of vWD is predominantly (90%) incompletely autosomal dominant. A few cases are recessively inherited (type IIc and type III) but sex-linked inheritance is not recorded.
• There is a quantitative deficiency of von Willebrand's factor (vWF), an adhesive glycoprotein secreted from endothelial surfaces and megakaryocytes. vWF is important for platelet adhesion and stabilization of factor VIII.
• vWD is characterized by abnormal bleeding of variable severity, predominantly from mucous membranes.
• Gastrointestinal bleeding, epistaxes and menorrhagia are frequent problems but petechiae are unusual.
• Bleeding tends to become less severe later in life.
• Investigations reveal a prolonged bleeding time and usually a defect of platelet adhesiveness. vWF immunoassay is the diagnostic test of choice.
• Cryoprecipitate contains all molecular forms of vWF and is more effective treatment for vWD than are factor VIII concentrates. There is a delayed secondary rise of the factor VIIIc levels after infusion of cryoprecipitate.

- DDAVP increases levels of vWF and is therapeutically useful. Repeated doses result in progressively less response.

LEE *et al.* (1993) pp.1432, 1450

12. The oculomotor nerve
ANSWERS: a b d

NOTES
- The oculomotor nucleus is situated in the midbrain just anterior to the cerebral aqueduct at the level of the superior and inferior colliculi.
- The fibres run through the medial longitudinal fasciculus and the red nucleus to emerge from the brainstem on the medial aspect of the crus cerebri.
- The oculomotor nerve (III) runs between the posterior cerebral and superior cerebellar arteries, in proximity to the posterior communicating artery. It then passes through the dura, over the free edge of the tentorium cerebelli, and into the lateral cavernous sinus. Here it lies close to the fourth and sixth nerves, and the ophthalmic branch of the trigeminal.
- The nerve supplies all the external ocular muscles, with the exception of the lateral rectus and superior oblique muscles. In addition it carries parasympathetic fibres.
- A complete third-nerve lesion results in ptosis (due to loss of parasympathetic supply of the levator palpebrae superioris), mydriasis, paralysis of accommodation and deviation of the eye laterally and downward (due to unopposed superior oblique and lateral rectus activity).
- Parasympathetic fibres lie peripherally in the nerve and ptosis with mydriasis may precede external ophthalmoplegia where nerve compression occurs.
- An isolated third-nerve palsy is associated with diabetes (probably a result of vascular disease); recovery usually occurs in 4–6 months.
- The sixth nerve runs close to the apex of the petrous temporal bone over which it may be stretched when raised intracranial pressure occurs and where it may be damaged by osteitis (Grandenigo's syndrome). It innervates the lateral rectus muscle.

WALTON (1993) p. 98

13. Ectopic adrenocorticotrophic hormone (ACTH) secretion
ANSWERS: a d e

NOTES
• Ectopic ACTH secretion is usually associated with a small-cell (oat-cell) carcinoma of the bronchus (60%). Less commonly, this syndrome may be associated with thymic tumours (15%), pancreatic carcinoma, usually islet cell (10%), bronchial carcinoids (4%) and, rarely, other tumours.

• Classical cushingoid features may develop (more often when the tumour is slow-growing). However the high ACTH levels produced by tumours and short history usually lead to a different presentation with generalized muscle weakness, mental abnormality, oedema (fluid retention), diabetes and skin pigmentation.

• The high steroid levels, resulting from ACTH stimulation, lead to a hypokalaemic alkalosis with sodium retention (due to mineralocorticoid action).

• Ectopic ACTH secretion is generally autonomous. Urinary steroid output is not increased after metyrapone administration, or the cortisol levels suppressed by dexamethasone. (However, partial responses may occur.) Elevated ACTH levels without diurnal variation are characteristic.

• The marked excess of urinary 17-ketosteroids compared with 17-hydroxysteroids seen in patients with carcinoma of the adrenal gland is not seen in the ectopic syndrome or Cushing's syndrome where the ratio is usually <3 : 1.

• Metyrapone, mitotane (o, p'-DDD) and aminoglutethimide may be used therapeutically to block adrenal steroid biosynthesis, if tumour resection or adrenalectomy is not possible. The long-acting somatostatin analogue octreotide has been observed to be effective.

• Metastasis to the adrenals frequently occurs in carcinomatosis due to bronchogenic carcinoma. However, hormonal deficiency as a result of replacement is very unusual.

DEGROOT *et al.* (1995) p. 2769

14. Myasthenia gravis

ANSWER: e

NOTES

• Myasthenia gravis is twice as common in women as in men. The peak age of onset is 20–30 years.

• There is a strong association with thyrotoxicosis.

• External ocular, bulbar and shoulder girdle are the most frequently involved muscles. Ptosis and diplopia are often early features. Muscle wasting is not seen in early cases but is common in long-standing cases.

• It is notable that tendon reflexes are normally brisk in myasthenia.

• Electromyogram (EMG) may demonstrate fatigability; however, clinical response to intravenous anticholinesterase (e.g. edrophonium chloride) usually establishes the diagnosis.

• Circulating antiacetylcholine receptor antibody is found in most adult-onset generalized active myasthenia gravis.

• Patients with medullary germinal centres on thymic histology, who are generally young females with human leucocyte antigen (HLA)-B8, DR3, respond well to thymectomy.

• Older patients with thymic involution generally have a poorer response to thymectomy.

• Patients with thymoma generally respond poorly to thymectomy.

• Anticholinesterases are the cornerstone of therapy. Prednisolone, sometimes with an immunosupressive agent, is frequently beneficial

• The Eaton–Lambert syndrome is a condition causing muscle weakness, predominantly of proximal muscles, associated with an underlying small-cell carcinoma of the bronchus (but up to 33% have no underlying carcinoma). Muscle power often improves after brief exercise. EMG shows increased evoked potentials after repeated galvanic stimulation (the opposite occurs in myasthenia gravis). Tendon reflexes are depressed.

• Anticholinesterase therapy is ineffective, but muscle power may improve after guanidine hydrochloride administration.

WALTON (1993) p. 645

15. Carbon dioxide retention

ANSWERS: c e

NOTES

• The arterial partial pressure of carbon dioxide ($Paco_2$) reflects alveolar ventilation. Hypoventilation results in an increased $Paco_2$. Pao_2 is influenced significantly by impairment of alveolar diffusion and ventilation–perfusion imbalance; it is a poor indicator of alveolar ventilation.

• Clinical features of carbon dioxide retention develop when the $Paco_2$ reaches 10.7 kPa (80 mmHg). They include tachycardia, hypertension, a bounding pulse with peripheral vasodilation (warm, sweaty extremities, injection of the eyes), muscle twitching, coarse tremor and confusion progressing to coma and death.

• Hypercapnia is associated with a raised intracerebral pressure. Headache is common and papilloedema may result.

• An elevated $Paco_2$ is associated with a reduction of blood and urinary pH. There is an increased urinary reabsorption of bicarbonate which results in an increased blood buffering capacity. Renal excretion of ammonium salts is increased but there is sodium retention.

• A $Paco_2$ of greater than 9.3 kPa (70 mmHg) has a direct depressive effect on the respiratory centre (situated in the reticular formation in the medulla). The hypoxic drive then becomes important.

• Hyperventilation is associated with a low $Paco_2$ and a respiratory alkalosis. If severe, tetany may result due to reduced levels of ionized calcium.

• Cerebral blood flow is sensitive to $Paco_2$ level. Flow may be greatly reduced when the $Paco_2$ is low.

• Left ventricular failure (pulmonary oedema) is associated with low or normal $Paco_2$ levels. Asthma is usually associated with hypoxia and hypocarbia except where forced expiratory volume in 1 s (FEV_1) is very severely reduced.

CROFTON & DOUGLAS (1989) pp. 528, 689

16. Classic phenylketonuria
ANSWERS: a c e

NOTES
• Classic phenylketonuria is a recessive condition which results from a deficiency of the hydroxylating enzyme for the conversion of phenylalanine to tyrosine.
• Classically, there is mental retardation, eczema, pigment dilution and seizures. Microcephaly occurs in 70% of untreated cases and epilepsy in 25%. Some 98% of untreated cases have an IQ of <70.
• Dietary reduction of phenylalanine intake reduces the mental defect. Early treatment is vital and maximal damage occurs by 4 years; thereafter introduction of a low-phenylalanine diet produces little improvement. After 10 years the diet can be relaxed without deterioration occurring.
• There is raised blood phenylalanine; the concentrations of many other amino acids in the blood are usually significantly reduced.
• The phenylalanine concentration is normal at birth but rises thereafter (more rapidly in males). Screening of the blood after 1 week identifies most cases. Urinary analysis at this stage is less accurate.
• Plasma tyrosine does not rise after a phenylalanine challenge in phenylketonuria (although administration of phenylalanine is detrimental and is contraindicated). Heterozygotes have a partial defect of phenylalanine metabolism, which may be identified after a phenylalanine challenge.

SCRIVER *et al.* (1989) p. 495

17. Subacute infective endocarditis
ANSWERS: a c d e

NOTES
• A low-grade fever is usual in SBE. Clubbing is associated but takes some weeks to develop and is now rare with early treatment. Mild splenomegaly is frequent and anaemia is universal. Change in the character of a pre-existing murmur is an unusual feature in subacute infection (but common in acute endocarditis).
• Petechiae and subungual splinter haemorrhages are associated, but may also occur in health and in other diseases. Osler's nodes (2–5 mm red tender nodules) are pathognomonic; they occur pre-

dominantly in pulp spaces. Janeway lesions (larger non-tender macules) and Roth spots (retinal 'soft' lymphocytic exudates) are also associated. Systemic or pulmonary emboli, depending on the site of infection, may occur, especially with fungal endocarditis.

• A· focal renal infarction, focal nephritis and diffuse glomerulone-phritis are very common, resulting in microscopic haematuria and proteinuria.

• SBE occurring in a patient with an atrial septal defect strongly suggests an ostium primum defect with infection of a cleft mitral valve. The ostium secundum type of defect is remarkably resistant to infection.

• Left-sided endocarditis is much more common (mitral 86%, aortic 55% of total) than right-sided endocarditis (tricuspid 20%, pulmonary 1%). Intravenous drug use is the commonest association with right-sided endocarditis.

• Blood culture is usually positive (>95% of cases). Arterial sampling does not result in a better positivity than does venous sampling.

• Rheumatoid factor is present in 50% of patients with endocarditis of >3 weeks' duration.

• The most frequent infecting organisms (in native valves in non-intravenous (IV) drug abusers) are currently:

(a) streptococci (50–70%)

(b) enterococci (10%)

(c) staphylococci (25%)

• In IV drug abusers with endocarditis *Staphyloccus aureus* is isolated in 60%, fungi represent <5%.

BRAUNWALD (1992) p. 1078

18. Phaeochromocytoma
ANSWER: e

NOTES

• 90% of phaeochromocytomas are sporadic (10% are familial), 90% occur in the adrenal (10% of tumours are extra-adrenal—usually intra-abdominal, situated or near sympathetic ganglia). Rarely tumours may occur in the bladder wall and symptoms may be provoked by micturition.

• 10% of spontaneous cases are bilateral (about 50% of familial cases are bilateral).

• Phaeochromocytomas may be familial and are associated with several related familial syndromes, the clinical features of which may include medullary carcinoma of the thyroid and hyperparathyroidism (multiple endocrine adenomatosis type 1 or MEN type 2, Sipple's syndrome), medullary carcinoma of the thyroid and multiple mucosal neuromas (MEN type 3). Phaeochromocytoma also occurs in some families with von Hippel–Lindau disease and occasionally in neurofibromatosis (<1% of cases).

• Between 2.4% and 14% of tumours are malignant.

• In phaeochromocytoma sustained hypertension occurs as frequently as does paroxysmal. Crises are associated with headache, anxiety, sweating and chest or abdominal pain. Headache, sweating and palpitations are the prominent symptoms, classically occuring in paroxysms. Orthostatic hypotension is a well-recognized feature.

• Diagnosis is established by vanillylmandelic acid (VMA) or metanephrine assay, urine being collected into strong acid.

• In most tumours the predominant granule is the one associated with noradrenaline whereas in the normal gland the predominant granule is adrenaline-containing.

• Chromogranin-A immunoreactivity can be identified in 100% of excised phaeochromocytomas and is increased in the blood of patients with these tumours.

• There is no association between tuberose sclerosis or the Sturge–Weber syndrome and phaeochromocytoma.

DEGROOT *et al.* (1995) p. 1853

19. Hyperthyroidism
ANSWERS: a b d

NOTES
• The commonest causes of hyperthyroidism are Graves' disease and toxic adenoma.

• Graves' disease includes ophthalmopathy, pretibial myxoedema and acropachy which are not associated with adenoma.

• In Graves' disease the thyroid is stimulated by an immunoglobulin (IgG). Thyroid stimulating antibody (TSAb) is present in over 90% of cases of Graves' disease but there is no correlation of the presence or titre of antibody with ophthalmopathy.

- A high level of TSAb in the third trimester of pregnancy forecasts neonatal hyperthyroidism.
- Characteristic clinical features include nervousness, heat intolerance, weight loss, sweating, palpitations and diarrhoea. A fine tremor is common.
- There is increased cardiac output, raised systolic blood pressure and a widened pulse pressure. Heart failure may result, especially in patients with underlying heart disease. Atrial fibrillation is a common feature in older patients.
- The skin is characteristically smooth, moist and erythematous. Pretibial myxoedema (which can occur at other sites, making the term dermopathy more suitable) is characterized by thickening of the skin, accentuation of hair follicles, erythema, itching and a clearcut edge to the lesion.
- Onycholysis is common in severe thyrotoxicosis. Thyroid acropachy may be associated with periosteal new bone formation.
- Menstrual disturbance is common (oligomenorrhoea is typical).
- Hypercalciuria is common while hypercalcaemia occurs infrequently, presumably both as a result of increased bone turnover.
- The concentration of red-cell 2,3-diphosphoglycine (2,3 DPG) is supranormal in thyrotoxicosis and the rate of synthesis of this compound has been seen to be significantly increased in response to thyroid hormones *in vitro*.

DEGROOT *et al.* (1995) p. 676

20. Classical mitral stenosis
ANSWERS: b d e

NOTES
- In mitral stenosis reflex pulmonary arteriolar vasoconstriction, in response to raised pulmonary venous pressure, results in reduced perfusion of basal regions of lung (when in the upright position); flow to upper regions is increased. This is the opposite of the normal stimulation and results in ventilation/perfusion inequality.
- In mitral stenosis vital capacity, forced expiratory flow rate and forced expiratory volume are reduced. The alveolar–arterial oxygen gradient is increased and the arterial oxygen tension falls. Dynamic compliance is markedly reduced.
- Accentuation of the first heart sound is characteristic and an

opening snap may be heard (unless the valve is calcified and immobile).

• An opening snap heard closely after the second sound is indicative of severe stenosis (due to high atrial pressure), as is a mid-diastolic murmur of long duration (intensity is not closely related to severity).

• The third heart sound results from rapid ventricular filling (as occurs in mitral incompetence); the obstructed valve prevents this in mitral stenosis.

• Haemoptysis is a common feature of mitral stenosis. The enlarged left atrium may rarely be associated with hoarseness due to left recurrent laryngeal nerve compression (Ortner syndrome).

• Thromboembolism is more common in older patients, those with low cardiac output and those with large left atrial appendages. A total of 80% of patients are in atrial fibrillation at the time that embolization occurs. Anticoagulation reduces the risk of embolization.

• A valve orifice of $<1.0 \, cm^2$ is considered critical stenosis and is associated with a gradient of about 20 mmHg; this is an indication for surgery in the presence of symptoms. Tachycardia increases the gradient as does increased flow (the transvalvular gradient is a function of the square of the flow).

BRAUNWALD (1992) p. 1007

21. Acyclovir

ANSWER: a

• Acyclovir inhibits herpes simplex I proliferation > herpes simplex II proliferation > herpes varicella-zoster.

• Epstein–Barr virus is only inhibited at very high levels and cytomegalovirus (CMV) proliferation is uninfluenced at clinically attainable concentrations.

• Viral thymidine kinase has about 200 times the affinity for acyclovir, as does mammalian thymidine kinase. Phosphorylation of acyclovir by mammalian thymidine kinase proceeds at a negligible rate.

• Acyclovir is predominantly excreted by the kidney with minimal metabolism.

• Cerebrospinal fluid (CSF) drug levels of acyclovir are about 50% of the corresponding blood level.

GILMAN et al. (1990) p. 1184

22. Tabes dorsalis
ANSWERS: a b c d e

NOTES
• Tabes dorsalis is seen much more frequently in males than in females (4 : 1). The first symptoms usually occur 8–12 years after syphilitic infection.
• There is degeneration of the intraspinal portion of the posterior nerve roots and of the sensory fibres of cranial nerves, especially of the fifth and ninth. Posterior column degeneration is associated and primary optic atrophy is common.
• Pain in the legs is usually the earliest symptom, classically localized stabbing 'lightning' pain. Paraesthesiae may also occur. Impairment of vibration and deep (tendon) pain sensation are early features.
• Pain perception is impaired over the side of the nose; medial border of the arm and forearm; the region of the chest between the nipples and costal margin; the lateral aspect of the leg; sole of the foot and the perianal region.
• Light touch and temperature sensation are usually unimpaired until the very advanced stages.
• Analgesia may predispose to Charcot joint and penetrating ulcer development.
• Ataxia is prominent and results from defective proprioceptive and spinocerebellar sense. The ataxia is worse in the dark or with the eyes closed—the basis of the Romberg test.
• Muscles are hypotonic and the reflexes depressed. Abdominal reflexes are frequently exaggerated. The bladder becomes atonic.
• Pupillary abnormality is common, but the complete Argyll Robertson pupil is a late manifestation. A moderate ptosis is common.
• There is a slight lymphocytosis in the CSF and a raised gamma-globulin. Reagin serology may occasionally be negative, but specific tests are almost invariably positive.
• Motor nerve conduction velocity is normal.

WALTON (1993) p. 295

23. Botulism
ANSWER: a

NOTES

• *Clostridium botulinum* is a Gram-positive spore-forming anaerobic organism; it may grow in preserved food when anaerobic conditions occur. Preserved (especially tinned) vegetables and fruit are particularly prone to infection.

• Several types of neruotoxin have been identified (A–G).

• The effects of botulism result from ingestion of the exotoxin which acts presynaptically, blocking acetylcholine release. Boiling for a few minutes destroys the toxin.

• Binding is irreversible and recovery occurs by sprouting of new terminal axons and formation of new neuromuscular junctions.

• The symptoms begin within 48 h of ingestion. Gastroenteritis may occur but constipation is more frequent. Pupillary dilation, ptosis, blurred vision and diplopia are usually the earliest features. There is usually no sensory loss and reflexes are generally preserved.

• Fever is not associated. There is extreme muscle fatigability and the electromyographic features resemble those of the Eaton–Lambert syndrome.

• Polyvalent antitoxin should be administered as early as possible. Antibiotic must be given if there is a chance of clostridial infection. Recovery is slow but usually complete.

WALTON (1993) p. 305

24. Thiamine deficiency
ANSWERS: a d e

NOTES

• Thiamine (vitamin B_1) is present in the germinal layer of rice and other cereals. Primary deficiency results from inadequate dietary intake; secondary deficiency may complicate chronic diarrhoea, alcoholism or liver disease.

• Thiamine deficiency interferes with pyruvate metabolism leading to an accumulation of pyruvate in the blood.

• High calorie intake increases the requirement for thiamine and predisposes to a state of deficiency.

• Deficiency usually results in a sensorimotor and autonomic neuropathy. There is axonal degeneration with secondary demyelination; sensory paraesthesiae; and muscle tenderness may be prominent and weakness profound ('dry' beriberi). In acute cases features may develop within 24–48 h.

• Features of 'wet' beri-beri may be associated and include tachycardia, a wide pulse pressure (hyperdynamic) and peripheral oedema, which may be very marked and associated with serous cavity effusions (high-output heart failure).

• The red-cell transketolase activity before and after the addition of thiamine pyrophosphate is the most sensitive test of deficiency.

WALTON (1993) p. 532

25. Dystrophia myotonica
ANSWERS: a c e

NOTES
• Dystrophia myotonica is characterized by weakness, wasting and myotonia of involved muscles. Facioscapular and distal limb muscles are predominantly affected.

• Associated features include frontal baldness, ptosis and a characteristic bland facies, cataracts, gonadal atrophy, mental deficiency or progressive dementia, cardiomyopathy and conduction defects, increased sweating and mildly abnormal thyroid function and glucose tolerance.

• 'Anticipation' (increasing severity of disease with succeeding generations) occurs in dystrophia myotonica apparently as a consequence of an increasing GCT repeat sequences in the protein kinase gene. (GCT repeat sequences in the protein kinase gene can be used to identify cases.).

• Pulmonary vital capacity is often impaired.

• Disordered smooth-muscle function leads to disordered oesophageal function and constipation.

• Immunoglobulins may be abnormal with excessive catabolism of IgG.

• Most patients show slow progressive deterioration. Cold and exercise tend to exacerbate myotonia.

• Procainamide is the most useful therapeutic agent. Phenytoin may be helpful.

• Testosterone may increase lean body mass but does not improve strength.

• Glutamylcysteine synthetase deficiency is a cause of adult spino-cerebellar degeneration, peripheral neuropathy and generalized amino-aciduria.

WALTON (1993) p. 632

26. Acute idiopathic thrombocytopenic purpura
ANSWERS: a c d

NOTES
• Most cases of acute idiopathic thombocytopenic purpura occur in children (most common 2–6 years) The sexes are equally affected in the acute form (females are affected more often than males in the chronic form).
• An IgG antiplatelet antibody is the responsible for the reduced platelet survival.
• There is diffuse petechial haemorrhage and ecchymoses. Mucous membrane bleeding is common, haemarthroses are rare. Cerebral haemorrhage occurs and accounts for most deaths in this condition. Marked splenomegaly is rare.
• The vast majority of cases make a spontaneous recovery within 2 months. Avoidance of aspirin is imperative. Prednisolone is recommended, although evidence that it influences the course of the disease is lacking. High-dose gammaglobulin inhibits platelet consumption by blocking macrophage Fc receptors. Platelet transfusion and emergency splenectomy may be required in severe cases.

LEE *et al.* (1993) p. 1330

27. Haemoglobinuria
ANSWER: c

NOTES
• Haptoglobin binds up to 1.4 g/l of free haemoglobin. Only when this is exceeded will free haemoglobin occur in the urine. This is only likely to occur when there is massive intravascular haemolysis.
• Causes include:
(a) paroxysmal nocturnal haemoglobinuria
(b) paroxysmal cold haemoglobinuria
(c) acute haemolytic crisis (sickle-cell, G6PD deficiency)

(d) autoimmune haemolytic anaemia

(e) toxins (methylchloride, chlorate, benzene, organic arsenicals)

(f) infections (malaria, blackwater fever, *Clostridium welchii*)

(g) extensive burns.

• Haemoglobinaemia is common in marathon runners, but is very rarely of such magnitude as to cause haemoglobinuria.

• Free haemoglobin in the glomerular filtrate is taken up by the renal tubular cells. These cells are shed and the haemosiderin may be identified in the urinary sediment.

• Ascorbic acid in the urine interferes with the biochemical reaction by which haemoglobin is detected in the urine.

HART (1985) p. 340

28. Which of the following statements about prostaglandins are true?

ANSWERS: a c e

NOTES

• Prostacyclin (PGI_2) is synthesized mainly by vascular endothelium and smooth muscle. It is a potent inhibitor of platelet aggregation but does not influence platelet adhesion or degranulation. PGI_2 also causes smooth-muscle relaxation with bronchodilatation and reduction of both systemic and peripheral vascular resistance.

• Prostaglandin Fs or PGFs (particularly $PGF_{2\alpha}$) cause marked pulmonary arteriolar muscle constriction (bronchoconstriction) and pulmonary hypertension. They have a strong oxytocic action.

• PGEs are powerful bronchodilators. They also exhibit oxytocic action (weaker than $PGF_{2\alpha}$)

• PGE_1 and PGE_2 both maintain ductus arteriosus patency in the newborn. (Prostaglandin inhibitors such as indomethacin have the opposite effect, enhancing closure.)

• PGEs and PGI_2 inhibit gastric acid secretion stimulated by feeding, histamine or gastrin.

• Leukotrienes contract most smooth muscles.

• Thromboxane A_2 is a powerful inducer of platelet aggregation and degranulation.

GILMAN *et al.* (1990) p. 600

29. Amyloidosis
ANSWERS: a c d

NOTES
• Primary amyloidosis is a disease of middle and advanced age, predominantly of men. Almost all cases have a monoclonal immunoglobulin in blood, urine or both. The amyloid protein AL (light-chain derivation) is associated.
• Features of primary amyloidosis include:
(a) sensorimotor peripheral neuropathy and autonomic neuropathy
(b) cardiomyopathy
(c) non-thrombocytopenic purpura
(d) macroglossia
(e) haemorrhagic diathesis (acquired factor X deficiency)
(f) proteinuria and eventually nephrotic syndrome
• Secondary amyloidosis complicates chronic inflammatory diseases including rheumatoid arthritis, ankylosing spondylitis, ulcerative colitris, etc. The amyloid protein AA is associated with secondary amyloidosis and familial Mediterranean fever.
• Rectal biopsy shows amyloid on Congo red staining in 75% of cases of systemic amyloidosis.
• Colchicine is generally effective in familial Mediterranean fever but is generally unhelpful in primary or secondary amyloidosis.

KELLEY *et al.* (1993) p. 1413

30. Neurofibromatosis of the von Recklinghausen type (NF1)
ANSWERS: b c d

NOTES
• NF1 accounts for >90% of cases of neurofibromatosis. It is an autosomal dominant condition with virtually complete penetrance but variable severity of manifestations (some patients may show only cutaneous pigmentation).
• About 50% of cases represent fresh mutations.
• Cutaneous pigmentation is almost invariable, represented by *café au lait* spots (usually with a regular outline, unlike the *café au lait* spots seen in Albright's syndrome).

• Cutaneous fibromas (soft swellings, pedunculated or sessile) are predominantly distributed over the trunk.
• Localized neurofibromas or 'plexiform neuromas' (neurofibromatosis with skin and subcutaneous tissue overgrowth) may occur.
• Melanocytic hamartomas of the iris (Lisch nodules) occur in all adult patients with NF1 and can be observed using slit-lamp examination.
• Acoustic neuromas and meningiomas probably do not occur with increased fequency in NF1 in comparison with the general population. Acoustic neuromas, often bilateral, are the central feature of NF2.
• Complications include spinal cord compression (a result of severe kyphoscoliosis or neuroma) and peripheral nerve compression.
• There is a recognized but rare association between neurofibromatosis and phaeochromocytoma (<1% of patients).

WALTON (1993) p. 427

31. Homozygous sickle-cell anaemia
ANSWERS: a b c d

NOTES
• In sickle-cell anaemia there is an abnormal haemoglobin–HbS. This haemoglobin has a reduced oxygen affinity and causes sickling when in the reduced state.
• Sodium metabisulphide leads to sickling in both the homozygous and heterozygous (sickle trait) disease when added to blood samples—this constitutes the most commonly used test of sickling.
• Sickle-cell anaemia is mainly seen among Africans and is also quite common in some areas of Greece.
• Homozygous patients are not anaemic at birth. Progressive anaemia occurs from about 3 months of age. The haemoglobin level is usually between 4 and 8%. There is reduced red blood cell survival (especially after prolonged sickling) and haemolysis. Anisocytosis and target cells are usual; a reticulocytosis and circulating nucleated red blood cells are often seen. Dactylitis is a feature in childhood. Frontal bossing of the skull results from widening of the diploë.
• Splenomegaly is usual in childhood. Repeating infarctions occur and splenomegaly is not a feature in adults. Loss of splenic function

with increased risk of overwhelming infection occurs early. Abdominal pain is very common in cases of sickle-cell anaemia.
• Chronic leg ulceration is a feature.
• There is often an impaired renal concentrating ability and episodic haematuria may occur.
• Haematological crises may be of the haemolytic or aplastic type. Aplastic crises may occur in all types of chronic haemolytic anaemia and often follow an acute infection.
• Hypoxia and infection may initiate crises; pregnancy also increases this liability.

LEE *et al.* (1993) p. 1068

32. Multiple myelomatosis
ANSWERS: d e

NOTES
• In myeloma the 'm' band on plasma electrophoresis means 'monoclonal'; it does not indicate that the paraprotein is IgM.
• The mean age of onset is about 60 years; back pain is very common but skull and limb pain are rare (although pathological fractures occur and cause pain); weight loss is common.
• Well-defined 'punched-out' lytic bone lesions are characteristic of myeloma; the lesions of secondary carcinoma are usually less well-defined. Since the process is almost purely lytic, alkaline phosphatase is usually not raised.
• Marrow replacement leads to pancytopenia. There is suppression of the level of normal functioning gammaglobulin and an increased liability to infection.
• The erythrocyte sedimentation rate (ESR) is usually raised, often to >100 mm/h.
• Hepatomegaly is often seen, splenomegaly less frequently.
• Renal damage is common as a result of hypercalcaemia, dehydration, deposition of light chains in the tubules, amyloid deposition and myeloma cell infiltration.
• In most cases the excess immunoglobulin is IgG (50–60%). It is IgA in about 25% of cases, light chains alone in about 20%. Other types are rare.
• Fewer than 2% are younger than 40 years at diagnosis.
• Calcitonin relieves bone pain, hypercalcaemia and aids healing of

lytic lesions (calcitonin binds to osteoclasts, inducing cyclic adenosine monophosphate (cAMP)-mediated depletion of intracellular calcium concentration which reduces bone-eroding activity).

• 40% of patients with chemotherapy-resistant and relapsing myeloma achieve second remission with glucocorticosteroids.

LEE *et al.* (1993) p. 2219
DEVITA, HELLMAN & ROSENBERG (1993) p. 1984

33. Inappropriate ADH secretion
ANSWERS: a c e

NOTES
• Cardinal features of the syndrome of inappropriate ADH secretion (SIADH) include hyponatraemia with low plasma osmolality and urine osmolality greater than plasma osmolality.
• A confident diagnosis of SIADH can only be made in the absence of hypotension, hypovolaemia or peripheral oedema in patients with normal adrenal and renal function.
• Conditions associated with inappropriate ADH production include:
(a) tumours: particularly small-cell carcinoma of the bronchus; more rarely others, including adenocarcinoma of the pancreas, lymphosarcoma
(b) pulmonary disease: pulmonary tuberculosis (vasopressin has been demonstrated in tuberculous lung tissue); pulmonary abscess and chest infection
(c) neurological conditions: head injury (skull fracture); subdural haematoma; subarachnoid haemorrhage; tuberculous and purulent meningitis; the Guillain–Barré syndrome; acute intermittent porphyria
(d) miscellaneous: treatment with chlorpropramide, cisplatin, phenothiazines.
• Treatment involves restricted fluid intake (500 ml/24 h). Demeclocycline treatment (600–1200 mg daily) may be effective. Normal saline or hypertonic saline infusions can be used in severe cases.
• The rate and magnitude of the increase of serum sodium appear to be risk factors for the development of the osmotic demyelination syndrome. Slow restoration of sodium levels is therefore recommended.

DEGROOT *et al.* (1995) p. 415

34. Polycythaemia rubra vera
ANSWERS: c

NOTES
• In PRV there is an increased red-cell mass (two to three times normal). The haemoglobin concentration and haematocrit are raised (unless there is associated haemorrhage). Iron deficiency changes may coexist.
• The leucocyte alkaline phosphatase activity is almost always normal or raised. The ESR is usually low (<5 mm/h). Both neutrophil leukocytosis and thrombocythaemia are commonly associated. B_{12} levels are increased predominantly due to increased transcobalamin III levels. Erythropoietin levels are not increased (in contrast to secondary polycythaemia).
• There is a predisposition to thrombosis but haemorrhage, especially from the gastrointestinal tract, is associated. Bleeding time is increased in only 20% of patients.
• The most common presenting symptoms are headaches, fullness in the head, dizziness and visual disturbances. Generalized pruritus (especially after a hot bath) is characteristic.
• A palpable spleen occurs in about 90% of cases, but it is not usually greatly enlarged.
• Termination of the disease as an acute myeloid leukaemia (AML) is unusual (<10% of cases), as is progression to myelofibrosis. Chromosomal abnormalities are seen in about 15% of cases at diagnosis.
• Phlebotomy aims to reduce the haematocrit below 46%. Phlebotomy alone results in an increased risk of thrombosis and concurrent treatment with antiplatelet agents in these patients results in a markedly increased risk of haemorrhage. Alkylating agents or P^{32} lead to an increased risk of malignant transformation over phlebotomy alone.

LEE *et al.* (1993) p. 1999

35. Cerebral tumours
ANSWER: e

NOTES
• Gliomas constitute about 40% of cerebral tumours, metastases about 20% and meningiomas about 10%; acoustic neuroma and pituitary adenoma comprise not >5% each.

- Meningiomas are more common in females.
- Meningiomas invade bone in about 20% of cases; however hyperostosis of the overlying bone may occur without invasion.
- The headache is often throbbing, occurs chiefly at night and in the early morning and persists for longer periods as the tumour enlarges. Manoeuvres which raise intracranial pressure (e.g. coughing, sneezing, vomiting, stooping and straining at stool) aggravate the headache.
- Subtentorial tumours may cause mainly suboccipital headache with radiation down the neck; neck flexion may aggravate this pain.
- Papilloedema tends to occur earlier and to be more severe when tumours are situated in the posterior fossa (e.g. cerebellar tumours) than when they are supratentorial.
- Epileptiform convulsions are more likely if the tumour is situated in or near the cerebral cortex. They are infrequent with tumours of the posterior fossa or brainstem. Epilepsy is more frequent with slow-growing than rapidly growing tumours. About 10% of those presenting with epilepsy aged >20 years are subsequently found to have a tumour (up to 40% where fits are focal).
- True vertigo is uncommon but severe vertigo in response to change of posture is a characteristic feature of fourth ventricular tumours (e.g. ependymoma).

WALTON (1993) p. 153

36. G6PD
ANSWERS: b c d

NOTES
- G6PD deficiency is associated with a bactericidal defect as a consequence of a subnormal neutrophil respiratory burst. Only patients with <5% G6PD activity suffer from recurrent bacterial infections.
- In most cases haemolysis occurs only after exposure to an oxidizing substance. Neonatal haemolysis and jaundice may occur.
- Drugs commonly implicated as the cause of haemolysis in patients with G6PD deficiency include:
(a) primaquine (and other 8-aminoquinolines)
(b) sulphonamides
(c) para-aminosalicylate

(d) nitrofurantoin

(e) dapsone.

• Some patients with G6PD deficiency develop acute haemolysis after ingestion of broad beans (*Vicia faba*).

• Oxidant damage leads to Heinz body formation. Spherocytosis is not a feature.

• Young cells have more G6PD activity than older cells.

• Hypoglycaemia is not a feature. In von Gierke's disease (G6PD deficiency), hepatomegaly, stunted growth and hypoglycaemia are characteristic.

SCRIVER *et al.* (1989) pp. 425, 2237, 2789

37. Brown-Séquard syndrome
ANSWERS: a b d e

NOTES

• The corticospinal tract is the most important motor tract; most fibres decussate in the medulla forming the lateral spinothalamic tract. A small proportion of fibres remain uncrossed and descend in the anterior corticospinal tract, which runs alongside the anterior median fissure.

• The sensory fibres conveying the sensation of posture (proprioception), the finer appreciation of tactile stimulation (cortical discrimination) and vibration sense have their cell bodies in the dorsal root ganglia. The fibres then pass to the ipsilateral posterior columns (without synapse in the posterior horn). Decussation of the posterior columns occurs in the lower brainstem.

• There is an orientation of the fibres within the posterior columns. Those fibres originating in the lower part of the cord ascend medially.

• Proprioceptive impulses also ascend to the cerebellum in the ipsilateral spinocerebellar tract (in the superficial part of the lateral column).

• Those fibres conveying the sensations of pain, temperature and crude tactile sensation synapse in the posterior horn of the spinal cord. The majority of fibres then decussate to ascend in the contralateral spinothalamic tract (in the anterior part of the lateral column).

• Those fibres which pass to the spinothalamic tract may ascend for some segments on the same side of the cord as they enter, before decussating. Fibres conveying pain sensation appear to run in the lateral aspect of the spinothalamic tract.

• Hemisection of the spinal cord (Brown-Séquard syndrome) results in ipsilateral loss of proprioception, vibration sense and fine tactile discrimination (posterior column damage) and ipsilateral upper motor neuron lesion below the lesion (corticospinal tract damage).

• There is contralateral analgesia and thermoanaesthesia (due to spinothalamic tract damage). The level of the cord lesion is generally some segments above that indicated by the upper level of the sensory loss (due to fibres ascending before decussation).

• There may be an ipsilateral lower motor neuron lesion, due to cord destruction at the level of the lesion.

WALTON (1993) p. 49

38. Henoch–Schönlein syndrome
ANSWERS: b c e

NOTES

• Henoch–Schönlein syndrome is characterized by a widespread necrotizing vasculitis (of arterioles and small capillaries) usually following an upper respiratory tract infection.

• Purpura, arthritis and cramping abdominal pain are the common features. Abdominal complications include intestinal haemorrhage and intussusception.

• Males are affected more frequently than girls. The peak incidence is between 4 and 11 years.

• IgA-containing immune complexes have been regularly demonstrated in the Henoch–Schönlein syndrome. Complement levels are usually normal.

• There is a non-thrombocytopenic purpura, mainly over the extensor surface of the buttocks and legs, which occurs in almost all cases and is usually the presenting feature. Macules or papules also occur, as may urticaria (especially of the face and legs). Lesions tend to occur in crops and may be provoked by abrading the skin.

• There is usually a transient non-migratory polyarthritis. Larger joints, especially of the lower limb, are predominantly involved.

• An acute proliferative glomerulonephritis (with haematuria and proteinuria) occurs in about 50% of cases. Occasionally there may be progression to chronic glomerulonephritis.

• The disease is usually self-limiting, especially in children. Corticosteroids may benefit joint and interstitial disease and prevent the progression to chronic renal disease.

KELLEY *et al.* (1993) p. 1087

39. Rubella
ANSWER: b

NOTES

• Babies with congenital rubella excrete virus for long periods—frequently 3 months or longer. They are highly infectious.

• Gammaglobulin, given soon after exposure, may reduce the incidence of clinical infection. However subclinical infection and viraemia can still occur and the fetus may become infected. The value of gammaglobulin to pregnant women exposed to rubella is disputed. The rise of antibody level after gammaglobulin injection is minimal; it does not therefore make subsequent serological tests difficult to interpret.

• A rising titre of IgG antibody (4 times) or the presence of IgM antibody is indicative of recent infection. Second subclinical infection can rarely occur some years after vaccination—there is then only a rise in the IgG antibody level (not IgM), and infection of the fetus does not seem to occur.

• Rubella is almost always a mild disease (unless congenital). Complications include arthritis (mainly involving small joints and occurring mostly, in about one-third of cases, in adult females), purpura and very rarely encephalitis.

• Rubella vaccination results in a 95% seroconversion rate. No case of congenital rubella syndrome has been reported in babies of women inadvertently vaccinated during pregnancy.

MANDELL, BENNETT & DOLIN (1995) p. 1242

40. Aminoaciduria
ANSWERS: a b d e

NOTES

• Normal individuals lose small quantities of glycine, glutamine, alanine, serine and histidine in the urine.

• Overflow of excess amino acid from the blood into the urine occurs in:

(a) inherited metabolic disorders (e.g. phenylketonuria, homocystinuria, maple syrup urine disease)

(b) severe chronic liver disease.

• Renal causes include:

(a) selective failure of tubular reabsorption (e.g. cystinuria, Hartnup disease)

(b) general tubular damage (Fanconi syndrome; e.g. cystinosis, Wilson's disease, galactosaemia, heavy metal poisoning, etc.).

HART (1985) p. 22

41. Ostium secundum atrial septal defect

ANSWERS: c d e

NOTES

• The majority of cases of atrial septal defect are of the secundum type (70%). The classical physical findings are fixed splitting of the second heart sound and a pulmonic flow murmur.

• Symptoms include dyspnoea and fatigue. However, cases are usually asymptomatic throughout childhood. Pulmonary hyperaemia predisposes to bronchitis. Haemoptysis is unusual in the absence of pulmonary hypertension.

• Atrial dysrhythmias, especially atrial fibrillation, occur in association with atrial septal defect. The incidence increases with age (onset before 20 years of age is unusual). Almost all (96%) adults aged 60 years or more with an atrial septal defect are symptomatic.

• Prolapse of the mitral valve has been demonstrated in up to 20% of cases of ostium secundum atrial septal defect.

• On electrocardiography a prolonged PR interval and incomplete right bundle branch block are common (less commonly, complete right bundle branch block). A left axis deviation is usual in association with ostium primum defects and a right axis deviation is common in association with ostium secundum defects. With the development of pulmonary hypertension the changes of right ventricular hypertrophy may be seen.

• Bacterial endocarditis at the site of a secundum defect very rarely occurs.

• Catheter evidence of a difference of 5 mmHg or more between the atria is against the diagnosis of atrial septal defect.

• A pulmonary blood flow in excess of 1.5 times the systemic flow is generally regarded as an indication for surgery (due mainly to the risk that pulmonary hypertension and Eizenmenger's syndrome may develop). Spontaneous closure is very rare.

BRAUNWALD (1992) pp. 906, 968

42. Psittacosis
ANSWERS: a e

NOTES

• *Chlamydia psittaci* is the aetiological agent of psittacosis. Virtually any species of bird can be infected, although psittacine birds are considered the major reservoir.

• 50% of cases occur in bird-owners. In 20% no history of contact with birds can be elicited.

• The incubation period is about 7–15 days. There is usually a fever, myalgia and headache. Dry cough is common.

• Endocarditis is a recognized complication.

• On the chest X-ray shadowing may be localized to one lobe, but is usually more diffuse.

• The sputum usually contains a few polymorphs. The peripheral blood white-cell count is usually relatively normal.

• Complement fixation testing is the usual method of establishing the diagnosis. There is no antigenic relationship to Proteus OX or cross-reactivity (in contrast to rickettsiae).

• Tetracycline is the treatment of choice. Penicillin is ineffective.

• Person-to-person spread is rare but can occur and there is a risk to laboratory workers handling specimens from patients or sick birds.

MANDELL, DOUGLAS & BENNETT (1995) p. 1440
CROFTON & DOUGLAS (1989) p. 309

43. Syringomyelia
ANSWERS: a b c d

NOTES

• The pathological features of syringomyelia are found mainly in the lower cervical and upper thoracic spinal cord.

- Decussating sensory fibres are involved first, resulting in dissociated sensory loss (loss of pain and temperature sensation with preservation of posterior column fine touch).
- Sensory loss characteristically begins in the ulnar aspect of the hand, forearm and arm and then progresses over the chest. Sensory loss may be unilateral or bilateral.
- The lesion progresses rostrally and the descending spinal tract and then the nucleus of the trigeminal nerve are involved causing dissociated sensory loss over the face. The loss progresses from behind the face forwards towards the nose.
- The medullary sympathetics may be involved causing a Horner's syndrome. Nystagmus is common.
- Muscle weakness and wasting occur (especially of the small muscles of the hand), due to anterior horn cell damage. Fasciculation is uncommon. With medullary extension the nucleus ambiguus may be involved, resulting in vagal and glossopharyngeal palsy. Occasionally the hypoglossal nucleus may be damaged, resulting in palsy of the tongue.
- Extensor plantar responses are found in most cases in the advanced stages. However, weakness and paralysis of the lower limbs are rare.
- Dissociated sensory loss can lead to the development of Charcot joints of the upper limb—more commonly of the shoulder, elbow and cervical spine than of the wrist and hand joints.
- The anterior–posterior diameter of the cervical vertebral canal is usually increased in cases of syringomyelia. A narrow canal is not associated.
- Syringomyelia is associated with a variety of deformities including spina bifida, the Arnold–Chiari malformation, cervical vertebral fusion (the Klippel–Feil syndrome), cervical ribs and kyphoscoliosis.

WALTON (1993) p. 506

44. Congenital adrenal hyperplasia (classical 21β-hydroxylase deficiency)

ANSWERS: a c d

NOTES
- 21β-Hydroxylase deficiency is the defect in >90% of cases of congenital adrenal hyperplasia. This condition occurs about once in 5000 live births.

• The reduced cortisol production stimulates pituitary ACTH secretion; this acts on the adrenal which, unable to increase cortisol output adequately, responds to stimulation by increased precursor production. These steroids have androgenic activity causing virilism in girls and precocious puberty in boys.

• 75% of patients with classic 21β-hydroxylase deficiency also have defective aldosterone synthesis. These patients become rapidly shocked in the neonatal period as a consequence of sodium loss. They have hyponatraemia, hyperkalaemia and plasma renin activity (PRA). Monitoring PRA assists management.

• 11β-Hydroxylase deficiency results in a similar clinical picture to 21β-hydroxylase deficiency but there is accumulation of 11-deoxycorticosterone which has a mineralocorticoid action resulting in hypertension.

• Treatment is by hydrocortisone replacement (which reduces the ACTH drive). Close monitoring is important; too much cortisone suppresses linear bone growth, while too little permits elevation of androgen levels which accelerate skeletal maturation. Mineralocorticoid is also indicated where salt loss is present.

• 21β-Hydroxylase deficiency can be treated *in utero* by administering dexamethasone to the mother. This results in normal external genital development in affected daughters.

SCRIVER *et al.* (1989) p. 1881

45. Sickle-cell trait
ANSWERS: c d

NOTES

• In sickle-cell trait there is no anaemia and red-cell survival is normal. Some 30–45% of the total haemoglobin is HbS. Iron deficiency and coexisting α-thalassaemia are associated with lower concentrations of HbS. Levels of HbA_2 are slightly increased.

• There is no splenomegaly. Growth, development and life expectancy are normal.

• Haematuria (due to renal papillary infarction) and splenic infarction are rare but well-recognized complications of patients with sickle-cell trait.

• Reduced ability to concentrate urine (hyposthenuria) is common.

• Sickling can be induced *in vitro*; it occurs more slowly than is the case in homozygous sickle-cell anaemia. Diagnosis is best established by haemoglobin electrophoresis.

LEE *et al.* (1993) p. 1084

46. Bile salts
ANSWERS: a b e

NOTES
• Bile salts are steroid metabolites of cholesterol. Cholic acid and choledeoxycholic acid are the major products.
• All of the bile salts excreted from the liver cell are conjugated with either glycine or taurine. Partial deconjugation occurs in the bowel due to the action of bacterial enzymes. Bacterial enzymes also result in the production of secondary bile salts.
• Bile salts are partially absorbed in the proximal small intestine, where most food is absorbed. There is active reabsorption of most of the bile salts in the terminal ileum.
• The vast majority of the excreted bile salt is reabsorbed and returns to the liver in the portal vein, where it is re-excreted (the enterohepatic circulation). Recirculation has been estimated to occur about six times per day. About 30% of the pool is lost per day. There is no absorption via the lymphatic system.
• The enterohepatic circulation may be interrupted by loss from a biliary fistula, binding to a binding agent (e.g. cholestyramine), impaired reabsorption due to ileal resection or disease or by bacterial overgrowth causing increased deconjugation and precipitation of the deconjugated salt.
• When there is excess loss of bile salts hepatic synthesis may increase up to 20 times the basal rate. Unsaturated fatty acids are absorbed better than saturated fatty acids in the presence of bile salt deficiency. Water-soluble medium-chain fatty acids are well absorbed in the presence of bile salt deficiency.
• Dihydroxy bile salts passing into the colon inhibit water absorption and may cause diarrhoea. Calcium binding to fatty acid results in increased levels of free oxylate and consequently increased urinary oxylate excretion.
• Chenodeoxycholic and ursodeoxycholic bile salts in large dose have been shown to promote gallstone dissolution (this is clinically effective in non-calcified, radiolucent stones, particularly those which are

95

small and are seen to float on the bile in the gallbladder). Deficiency of bile salts promotes gallstone formation.

• Blood bile acid levels are sensitive indicators of liver disease, particularly portosystemic shunting. Cerebrotendinous xanthomatosis is a result of a recessively inherited deficiency of choledeoxycholic acid.

SLEISENGER & FORDTRAN (1993) pp. 985, 1791, 1848

47. Systemic lupus erythematosus
ANSWER: all incorrect

NOTES
• SLE is much more common in females (9 : 1). Some 65% present aged between 16 and 55 years.
• Fibrinoid necrosis of small arteries and arterioles is the characteristic pathological finding.
• An erythematosus 'butterfly' rash occurs in about 50% of cases. There may be sensitivity to sunlight, urticaria, vasculitis (including livedo reticularis and vasculitic leg ulcers) and alopecia (in >60%), which is usually patchy in distribution.
• Arthralgia is almost universal. Small joints are predominantly involved; arthritis is generally non-erosive. Ulnar deviation at the metacarpophalangeal joints with subluxations may occur with chronic disease.
• Clinical renal involvement (glomerulitis/glomerulonephritis) occurs in 50%. Proteinuria occurs at some time in 78% of patients. Renal lesions include focal proliferative, diffuse proliferative, membranous and mesangial glomerulonephritis.
• Neurological features include seizures, hemiplegia or other focal signs, cranial nerve lesions, cerebellar signs, aseptic meningitis and occasionally peripheral neuropathy. The electroencephalogram frequently shows diffuse abnormality.
• Lymphadenopathy may occur (50%), especially during exacerbations. Splenomegaly occasionally occurs (20%).
• A normochromic normocytic anaemia is common. An autoimmune haemolytic anaemia occurs in 6–15%. Leukopenia is common; thrombocytopenia may occur.

KELLEY et al. (1993) p. 1017

48. Primary hyperaldosteronism (Conn's syndrome) due to adrenal adenoma

ANSWERS: a b e

NOTES

• Aldosterone enhances renal sodium reabsorption, but after a few days the kidney escapes from this effect and oedema does not develop (in the absence of heart failure).

• Primary hyperaldosteronism may result from adrenal hyperplasia, adrenal adenoma or adrenal carcinoma. Adrenal adenoma is the commonest cause (66% of cases). Calcification is common in adrenal carcinomas. Ectopic aldosterone secretion from tumours is extremely rare.

• Renal potassium loss continues when aldosterone secretion/administration is prolonged (i.e. there is no escape from this action). Potassium-wasting diuretic therapy tends to exacebate or reveal the hypokalaemia.

• Mild hypertension is characteristic. Muscle weakness may be a feature while intermittent paraesthesia and tetany or periodic paralysis (possibly more common in Chinese patients) occur infrequently.

• Hypokalaemic alkalosis leads to polyuria (as a result of reduced renal concentrating ability) and polydipsia.

• The plasma renin level is low in primary hyperaldosteronism.

• The presence of hypokalaemia in an untreated hypertensive patient is an indication for investigation of the renin–angiotensin–aldosterone axis. If the plasma potassium level is below 3.0 mmol/l this should be increased before testing.

• Plasma aldosterone should be measured at a fixed time of day in a standard posture (usually lying). Plasma aldosterone levels characteristically fall on standing in patients with adenoma while an increase is seen after standing in patients with hyperplasia. A high aldosterone : renin ratio has been used to indicate the diagnosis of primary hyperaldosteronism.

DEGROOT (1995) p. 1775

49. Pseudohypoparathyroidism, type I
ANSWERS: a c

NOTES

• PHP is a rare familial disorder (probably inherited as an autosomal dominant with variable expression), in which there is end-organ unresponsiveness to parathyroid hormone.

• In PHP type I there is deficient urinary cAMP excretion in response to PTH while in PHP type II there is a normal cAMP response to PTH despite impaired phosphaturic response (PHP type II probably represents a number of heterogeneous conditions).

• The biochemical findings resemble those seen in hypoparathyroidism with hypocalcaemia (due to impaired calcium mobilization from bone, reduced intestinal absorption and increased urinary calcium loss) and hyperphosphataemia (consequent on a reduced phosphaturic response in the kidney). Hypocalcaemia results in clinical tetany (onset usually about 8 years).

• Other features include subcutaneous calcification (rare in acquired hypoparathyroidism), short stature, obesity, brachydactyly (especially of the fourth and fifth metacarpals), impaired glucose tolerance and mental retardation.

• Pseudopseudohypoparathyroidism shows similar somatic features but normal biochemical findings. Occurrence of pseudopseudohypoparathyroidism in the same families as PHR has been reported and may represent incomplete genetic expression.

DEGROOT (1995) p. 1136

50. Vitamin B_{12} deficiency
ANSWERS: a b c d e

NOTES

• Vitamin B_{12} (cobalamin) is metabolized in the body to 5′-deoxyadenosyl-1 cobalamin. This is the coenzyme in the conversion reaction of methylmalonyl CoA to succinyl CoA (urinary methylmalonyl CoA excretion is increased in the presence of vitamin B_{12} deficiency).

• Methylcobalamin is a cofactor (with folic acid) in the methylation of homocystine to form methionine.

• Results of vitamin B_{12} deficiency include peripheral neuropathy–paraesthesiae of the extremities is usually the earliest symptom.

There may be a 'glove-and-stocking' anaesthesia which develops proximally.
• Combined degeneration of the cord may develop with predominant involvement of the dorsal columns and corticospinal tracts. Postural sensitivity and vibration sense are almost invariably impaired. Weakness and spasticity or sensory ataxia (a result of spinocerebellar tract and posterior column damage) may predominate in the lower limbs.
• Bilateral primary optic atrophy is associated. Tobacco amblyopia may be caused by the traces of cyanide in tobacco smoke interfering with vitamin B_{12} utilization; it is treated with hydroxycobalamin.
• Confusion, memory loss, depression, dementia or psychosis may all occur and respond to replacement therapy.
• Neuropathy secondary to vitamin B_{12} deficiency may rarely occur in the absence of anaemia.

WALTON (1993) p. 537

51. Vitamin D deficiency
ANSWERS: a b c d e

NOTES
• Rickets and osteomalacia result in moderate hypocalcaemia, hypophosphataemia and increased serum alkaline phosphatase activity.
• Associated bone involvement is predominantly of the appendicular rather than the axial skeleton.
• Onset during infancy may lead to craniosynostosis, flattening of the pelvis and incomplete greenstick fractures of the lower limbs.
• Prominent features during childhood include costochondral swelling (rachitic rosary), recession at the diaphragm (Hutchinson's grooves) and a protuberant sternum. There is growth retardation and bone pain with cartilaginous enlargement and deformity at sites of endochondrial ossification.
• Proximal muscle weakness is a feature and hypocalcaemia of sufficient severity to cause tetany may occur.
• Radiological features include generalized bone rarefaction with increased trabecular markings. There may be local areas of excessive rarefaction resembling fractures (Looser's zones, pseudofractures). Widened osteoid seams are the characteristic histological finding.
• Causes of osteomalacia and rickets include:
(a) dietary vitamin D deficiency

(b) absorption
(c) chronic renal disease
(d) renal tubular disease
(e) familial hypophosphataemic rickets
(f) hypophosphatasia
• Anticonvulsant therapy may interfere with vitamin D metabolism and lead to rickets and osteomalacia.

DEGROOT (1995) p. 990

52. β-Thalassaemia major
ANSWERS: a e

NOTES
• In β-thalassaemia major there is a marked hypochromic microcytic anaemia. Red-cell survival is reduced, target cells are seen and circulating nucleated red cells are always present. The reticulocyte count is usually low.
• Fetal haemoglobin (HbF) is usually raised to between 30 and 60%. The HbA_2 concentration is variable but is usually within the normal range.
• There is erythroid hyperplasia of the marrow which may cause cortical thinning of the long bones and pathological fracture.
• There is usually a mild hyperbilirubinaemia (reflecting haemolysis). Serum iron is usually raised and iron-binding capacity saturated. Haemosiderosis, often with features of haemochromatosis, is common.
• A raised HbA_2 concentration is characteristic in the β-thalassaemia trait (unless there is associated iron deficiency) and HbF concentration is not elevated.
• Prenatal diagnosis is possible with fetal blood sampling or gene probe analysis of amniotic fluid cells.

LEE et al. (1993) p. 1118

53. Chronic autoimmune adrenal insufficiency
ANSWERS: b c d e

NOTES
• Autoimmune adrenal insufficiency is the commonest cause of

primary adrenal insufficiency in the western world (tuberculosis is a more common cause in the Third World).

• In 50% of cases there is evidence of a polyglandular autoimmune syndrome.

• Polyglandular autoimmune syndrome type I is a rare recessive disorder occuring in childhood which includes adrenal insufficiency, hypoparathyroidism and mucocutaneous candidiasis.

• Polyglandular autoimmune syndrome type II is more common, has a mean onset of 24 years, and includes adrenal insufficiency, autoimmune thyroid disease and diabetes mellitus. Inheritance appears to be autosomal dominant.

• Muscle weakness, anorexia and fatigue are the major complaints of patients with adrenal insufficiency. Orthostatic hypotension is characteristic.

• In primary adrenal insufficiency ACTH levels are raised and resulting hyperpigmentation particularly involves skin folds, areas of trauma and mucous membranes (in contrast, the pigmentation of haemochromatosis rarely affects mucous membranes). Areas of vitiligo may be associated and do not become hyperpigmented.

• There is frequently normochromic normocytic anaemia and relative lymphocytosis with increased eosinophil count. Hyponatraemia with hyperkalaemia is characteristic.

DEGROOT (1995) p. 1731

54. Phrenic nerve
ANSWERS: d e

NOTES
• The phrenic nerve is a branch of the cervical plexus. It arises principally from the ventral primary ramus of the fourth cervical nerve (it also receives contributions from the third and fifth cervical nerve).

• The nerve passes downward on the posterolateral aspect of the internal jugular vein under the sternocleidomastoid muscle.

• The phrenic nerve leaves the neck and enters the thorax by passing in front of the subclavian artery and behind the vein. On the left it crosses the thoracic duct and the arch of the aorta before crossing in front of the root of the lung. On the right the nerve runs in close relationship to the superior vena cava, in front of the root of the lung.

• The nerves then run over the pericardium, through the diaphragm and innervates the diaphragm from the inferior surface.

• The phrenic nerves also convey afferent fibres from the mediastinal and diaphragmatic pleura, the pericardium, diaphragmatic peritoneum, liver and gallbladder. Stimulation of these afferent fibres results in referred pain in the cutaneous area supplied by the fourth cervical nerve (and to a lesser extent the third and fifth).

WALTON (1993) p. 580

55. Acromegaly (hypersomatotrophism)
ANSWERS: c d e

NOTES

• Growth hormone exerts its growth-promoting action by way of insulin-like growth factors (IGF-I and IGF-II).

• In acromegaly there is soft-tissue and bone overgrowth, including a thickened heel pad which may be measured on X-ray. Laryngeal thickening gives rise to the characteristic deep voice. The sella turcica may be shown to be enlarged on X-ray in the majority of cases (about 90%).

• Glucose tolerance is impaired in 30–40% of cases of acromegaly. Clinical diabetes occurs in 10–20%.

• Hypertriglyceridaemia occurs in 19–44% of acromegalic patients (lipoprotein lipase activity is reduced).

• 1,25-Hydroxycholecalciferol levels are increased, resulting in increased gut calcium absorption. Serum calcium is normal but urinary calcium excretion is increased. There is a 6–12% incidence of urolithiasis.

• Prolactin levels are increased in 15–40% of cases of acromegaly.

• Hypoadrenocorticism is very rare and associated with the most aggressive tumours.

• Dopaminergic drugs (L-dopa, bromocriptine) increase growth hormone secretion in normal individuals; however in most patients with acromegaly growth hormone levels are paradoxically decreased by these drugs.

• Octreotide results in a reduction of both growth hormone and IGF-I levels in 80–90% of cases of acromegaly. Tumour size is reduced in about 50% of cases.

DEGROOT (1995) p. 303

56. Hyperlipidaemia of cholestasis

ANSWERS: d e

NOTES

• When cholestasis is prolonged serum phospholipids and free cholesterol rise. (Cholesterol esters and neutral fat remain at reasonably normal levels).

• An abnormal low-density lipoprotein (lipoprotein X) is associated and contains a high proportion of free cholesterol and lecithin. High-density lipoprotein is reduced.

• LCAT deficiency is a marked feature of both intrahepatic and extrahepatic cholestasis.

• Flat planar xanthomas are characteristic and occur in palmar creases, below the breast and on the neck, chest and back. Tuberous xanthomas occur later, characteristically on extensor surfaces, on pressure points and in scars. Tendinous xanthomas are rarely seen.

• Xanthomata do not occur unless cholestasis is of longer than 3 months' standing.

• The incidence of coronary arterial disease does not appear to be significantly increased by long-standing cholestasis and the associated hyperlipidaemia.

• Cholestyramine lowers serum bile acid and cholesterol levels. Xanthomata regress and pruritus is relieved in patients with cholestasis.

SHERLOCK & DOOLEY (1993) pp. 24, 225

57. Herpes simplex encephalitis

ANSWERS: a d e

NOTES

• Herpes simplex encephalitis affects all age groups (33% aged <20 years), most commonly due to viral reactivation.

• It usually occurs in previously fit (not immunocompromised) patients who already have circulating antibody from previous herpes simplex infection. The rate of herpes simplex encephalitis is not increased in immunocompromised patients.

• The vast majority of herpes simplex encephalitis is caused by herpes simplex virus type 1 (HSV-1).

• Herpes simplex encephalitis is rarely associated with recurrent herpes labialis.

• Herpes simplex encephalitis is characterized by acute severe necrotizing encephalitis, particularly of medial temporal and subfrontal regions.

• A prodromal period of 4–10 days is common with malaise, fever, headache and irritability. Signs include meningism, depressed consciousness and seizures (focal or generalized). Focal signs occur in most patients (87%).

• Herpes simplex encephalitis cannot be diagnosed on serum antibody tests but identification of herpes simplex by polymerase chain reaction is diagnostic.

• Mortality rates range from 40 to 70% (more in those unconscious on presentation) in untreated cases. Early acyclovir treatment reduces mortality to about 30%. Considerable disability is common in survivors.

WALTON (1993) p. 325

58. Conjugated hyperbilirubinaemia
ANSWERS: a b c d

NOTES
• Conjugation of bilirubin increases its water-solubility.
• Raised levels of serum conjugated bilirubin with relatively normal transaminase levels occur with cholestasis.
• Cholestasis is a feature of the sensitivity reaction to various drugs, including chlorpromazine, other phenothiazines, erythromycin, estolate and imipramine. Dose-related cholestasis complicates steroid (usually 17-alkylated steroid) therapy.
• Both viral and alcohol-induced hepatitis may have predominantly cholestatic features. Cholestasis may precede the hepatocellular picture.
• Primary biliary cirrhosis and sclerosing cholangitis are associated with cholestatic jaundice.
• There is impaired conjugated bilirubin excretion and hyperbilirubinaemia in the Dubin–Johnson and Rotor syndromes (alkaline phosphatase levels are not elevated).
• In Gilbert's syndrome there is an unconjugated mild hyperbilirubinaemia (common in 2–5% of the population).

SHERLOCK & DOOLEY (1993) pp. 119, 342

59. Gaucher's disease

ANSWERS: a c d

NOTES

• In Gaucher's disease there is tissue glucosylceramide accumulation in the reticuloendothelial system as a result of low glucocerebrosidase activity. (Sphingomyelin accumulation occurs in Niemann–Pick disease).

• Chronic (non-neuropathic) Gaucher's disease is characterized by marked splenomegaly, hepatomegaly and erosions of the cortices of long bones and the pelvis (which may cause pathological fracture). Expansion of the cortex of the lower femurs is frequent. Hypersplenism with anaemia, leukopenia and thrombocytopenia is a frequent complication. Splenectomy is often required.

• Acute neuropathic Gaucher's disease is rare. There is rapidly progressive neurological degeneration and death.

• Inheritance is recessive. Cases have been reported from most races; however it is most frequent among Ashkenazi Jews.

• A raised serum acid phosphatase activity (not tartrate-labile) is frequently associated with Gaucher's disease.

• Identification of deficient glucocerebrosidase activity in amniotic fluid cells or chorionic villi permits prenatal diagnosis.

• Heterozygotes tend to have low enzyme activity, but carrier detection is unreliable (failing to identify up to 20% of known heterozygotes).

• The cherry-red spot characteristic of some sphingolipidoses and mucolipidoses does not occur in Gaucher's disease.

SCRIVER et al. (1989) p. 1677

60. Cirrhotic ascites

ANSWER: b

NOTES

• The aetiology of ascites complicating liver disease is multifactorial but portal hypertension is important.

• The ascitic fluid in cirrhosis is transudate. The protein content is rarely greater than 20 g/l.

• Ascites complicating cirrhosis is associated with sodium retention (reduced urinary sodium excretion). The serum sodium level is usually slightly low but the total body sodium is increased.

• Sodium retention results from secondary aldosteronism (with raised aldosterone and renin levels).

• ANF levels are usually increased in those with ascites (but does not result in net renal sodium loss).

• Serum potassium is normal or slightly reduced, but total body potassium is reduced.

• A pleural effusion, usually right-sided (67%), is occasionally seen (6% of cases of ascites due to cirrhosis). Isolated left-sided effusions should suggest other additional pathology.

• Gram-negative infection occurs spontaneously in about 8% of patients with ascites, usually (up to 80%) due to Gram-negative aerobic bacteria. Infection is more likely in those with ascites with a low protein content (<10 g/l)

SHERLOCK & DOOLEY (1993) p. 129

61. Chronic active autoimmune hepatitis
ANSWER: all incorrect

NOTES
• Chronic active autoimmune hepatitis is characterized by an inflammatory mononuclear cell infiltrate predominantly in the portal zone. Most infiltrating cells are B lymphocytes or helper T lymphocytes (few suppressor/cytotoxic lymphocytes). Piecemeal necrosis and destruction of the liver architecture occur in severe cases.

• Chronic active hepatitis is more common in females (8 : 1); half present before 20 years of age. There is an association with the HLA B8 DR3 tissue type (who tend to present earlier with more severe disease and to relapse more frequently).

• Smooth-muscle antibody is present in about 70% of cases and ANA in about 80% (homogeneous pattern). Antimitochondrial antibody is usually absent or present only in low titre. LE-cells occur in about 15% of cases.

• Polyclonal hypergammaglobulinaemia is usual.

• 25% of cases present as an acute hepatitis; rarely a deep cholestatic jaundice may occur. Some cases run an anicteric course.

• The liver is enlarged in the early stages but becomes shrunken and cirrhotic as the disease progresses. Spider naevi are almost invariable.

• Keratoconjunctivitis sicca, leucopenia and thrombocytopenia are associated. Autoimmune haemolytic anaemia, non-destructive mi-

gratory polyarthritis, splenomegaly (in the absence of portal hypertension) and lymphadenopathy may also be associated.
• Corticosteroid treatment reduces symptoms and prolongs life. The 10-year survival is 63%.

SHERLOCK & DOOLEY (1993) p. 293

62. Primary biliary cirrhosis
ANSWERS: b d e

NOTES
• Mitochondrial antibodies (specifically to the M2 antigen which is a component of the pyruvate dehydrogenase complex of mitochondrial enzymes) occur in virtually 100% of cases with ANF in 27%.
• The majority of cases are female (90%). There is usually insidious onset of pruritus without jaundice. Jaundice preceding pruritus is very unusual.
• The liver is usually enlarged and firm. Skin pigmentation develops. The sicca syndrome is a frequent association (up to 75% of cases). Finger clubbing is associated. Xanthomata usually develop, sometimes with neuropathy.
• Fleshy lymphadenopathy at the porta hepatis is common (81% on computed tomographic or CT scanning), which may cause diagnostic difficulty. Widespread tissue granulomas (resembling those seen in sarcoidosis) may occur. The Kveim test is negative.
• An association with CRST syndrome is documented (calcinosis, Raynaud's phenomena, sclerodactyly, telangiectasia).
• Corticosteroids result in less pruritus and lower plasma liver enzyme levels but markedly enhance osteodystrophy and are therefore contraindicated. Supplementation by fat-soluble vitamins and calcium is required. Transplantation is effective in selected patients with advanced disease.

SHERLOCK & DOOLEY (1993) p. 236

63. Hereditary haemorrhagic telangiectasia
ANSWERS: b e

NOTES
• Hereditary haemorrhagic telangiectasia (Rendu–Osler–Weber

107

disease) is characterized by recurrent episodes of bleeding from congenitally abnormal thin-walled blood vessels.

• Inheritance is autosomal dominant.

• Telangiectasias are usually visible on the mucosa of the nose, mouth and tongue. Epistaxis is by far the most common complaint. Lesions are also often scattered over the skin of the face and pulps of fingers.

• The number and size of lesions tend to increase with age.

• Though a few telangiectasias often occur in the gastrointestinal tract, they may be diffusely distributed throughout and are associated with haemorrhage.

• Arteriovenous malformations increase with frequency with age. Pulmonary arteriovenous malformations are present in 90% of patients older than 60 years.

• Oestrogens induce metaplasia of the nasal mucosa and may usefully reduce the frequency and severity of epistaxes. Embolization is the preferred treatment for arteriovenous malformations.

LEE *et al.* (1993) p. 1379

64. Homocystinuria
ANSWERS: a b c d e

NOTES

• Cystathionine β-synthetase deficiency is the commonest cause of homocystinuria. Other causes include inherited or acquired deficiencies of methyltetrahydrofolate-homocystine methyltransferase.

• Plasma methionine and homocystine levels are elevated and homocystine is excreted in urine. Plasma cystine concentration is much reduced.

• Inheritance is recessive (Marfan's is dominant).

• Some features of homocystinuria resemble those of Marfan's syndrome, including ectopia lentis, arachnodactyly and kyphoscoliosis. In addition there is generalized osteoporosis, mental retardation (frequently), a malar flush, livedo reticularis and thromboses of intermediate-size arteries and veins (with pulmonary embolism)–none of which are features of Marfan's syndrome.

• Dissecting aortic aneurysm, which may occur in Marfan's syndrome, has not been reported in homocystinuria.

• The urinary cyanide–nitroprusside test serves as a screening test (also positive in cystinuria).

• Many cases respond to pyridoxine supplementation (probably those with some residual cystathionine β-synthetase activity). Prognosis in those cases which are pyridoxine-responsive is better than in those who are not responsive.

SCRIVER *et al.* (1989) p. 698

65. Diabetes mellitus
ANSWERS: a b c d e

NOTES
• Circulating cytoplasmic islet cell antibodies (ICA) and insulin autoantibodies (IAA) are present in approximately 80% of patients with type I diabetes at the time of diagnosis.
• Antibodies to the 64 kDa antigen (GAD) are found in 95% of patients with insulin-dependent diabetes mellitus (IDDM), but disappear over the next few years in most patients.
• Most cases (type IA) appear to have a genetic predisposition to IDDM; 10% (type IB) of cases have associated autoimmune endocrine disease.
• >90% of patients with IDDM younger than 30 years of age at onset are HLA-DR3 or HLA-DR4-positive.
• HbA_{1c} results from the addition of a hexose group to the N-terminal valine of the normal HbA_1 chain. The rate of formation of HbA_{1c} is proportional to the time–average concentration of glucose within the erythrocyte. When blood glucose is well-regulated, HbA_{1c} levels reduce after a period of 5–6 weeks.
• HbA_{1c} levels are not as sensitive as the oral glucose tolerance test in detecting diabetes or impaired glucose tolerance.

DEGROOT *et al.* (1995) p. 1411

66. Hepatitis C
ANSWERS: a b d e

NOTES
• Antihepatitis C antibody (antihepatitis C virus or anti-HCV) is detected in 0.5–1% of blood donors worldwide. Heat treatment of blood products destroys HCV. Anti-HCV is found much more commonly in human immunodeficiency virus (HIV) and HBV antibody-positive patients.

• HCV is much less infectious than is HBV.
• HCV has an incubation period of 5–12 weeks. Only 25% of patients become jaundiced. At 1 year 50% have chronic hepatitis and 20% progress to cirrhosis.
• In chronic hepatitis there is a fluctuating course with marked variation in transaminase levels over time (but rarely greater than six times normal).
• Portal hypertension is rare and varices are a late feature.
• An association of hepatocellular carcinoma with HCV infection is recognized
• Interferon treatment (3 million units, three times weekly for 1 year) effectively reduces transaminase levels but relapse rates are high.

SHERLOCK & DOOLEY (1993) pp. 283, 313

67. Abetalipoproteinaemia
ANSWERS: b c d

NOTES
• Abetalipoproteinaemia is a rare recessive disorder in which there is an inability to manufacture low-density lipoprotein (LDL). Chylo-micron formation is defective.
• Characteristic features include steatorrhoea, failure to thrive, low serum lipid concentrations (both cholesterol and triglycerides) and abnormal red blood cell morphology (acanthocytosis) presenting in the first 2 years of life.
• In later childhood ataxia, intention tremor, nystagmus, athetosis, muscle weakness and depressed tendon reflexes are seen.
• Later in childhood ataxia, intention tremor, nystagmus, athetosis, muscle weakness and depressed tendon reflexes occur.
• Intelligence is usually normal.
• Retinitis pigmentosa is a late manifestation.

SCRIVER et al. (1989) p. 1145

68. Glycosuria
ANSWERS: a b c d e

NOTES
• Glycosuria is the hallmark of diabetes mellitus. Impaired glucose

tolerance curve may occur in thyrotoxicosis and after gastrectomy.

• Raised adrenaline levels, as may occur in phaeochromocytoma, anxiety states and strenuous exercise, can cause the blood sugar level to rise above the renal threshold.

• Gross cerebral injury or haemorrhage may cause glycosuria.

• Severe infection, especially staphylococcal, impairs glucose tolerance.

• Gross hepatic dysfunction usually leads to hypoglycaemia; however a lag glucose tolerance curve may occur with glycosuria.

• Reduced renal threshold for glucose, as occurs during pregnancy, predisposes to glycosuria.

HART (1985) p. 310

69. Idiopathic hypoparathyroidism
ANSWERS: a c d

NOTES

• Idiopathic hypoparathyroidism includes those forms of hypoparathyroidism not due to surgery or other acquired causes. Familial isolated hypoparathyroidism is solitary in its clinical manifestation and is not associated with other endocrine abnormalities (as in polyglandular failure type I) or developmental abnormalities (as in DiGeorge syndrome). Only a minority of cases of isolated hypoparathyroidism appear to have a familial basis.

• Features include hypocalcaemia, which is associated with increased neuromuscular excitability or tetany, paraesthesiae (especially perioral or distal) and convulsions.

• Idiopathic hypoparathyroidism is usually associated with a normal alkaline phosphatase level.

• In idiopathic (or postsurgical) hypoparathyroidism, injection of PTH results in an increased urinary phosphate and cAMP excretion (in contrast to the situation in pseudohypoparathyroidism, PHP).

• Levels of PTH are usually normal or increased in PHR and vitamin D deficiency but are low in hypoparathyroidism.

• Urinary calcium excretion is low in hypoparathyroidism.

• Transient hypoparathyroidism due to magnesium deficiency may occur in patients with a history of alcoholism, diuretic use or malabsorption syndrome.

DEGROOT *et al.* (1995) p. 1127

70. Thrombolytic treatment for myocardial infarction
ANSWERS: a b

NOTES

• Intravenous recombinant tissue plasminogen activator (rt-PA) has been shown to result in better early patency rate when compared to intravenous streptokinase. However neither the GISSI[2] (Gruppo Italiano Per lo Studio della Streptochinasi nell' Infarcto Miocardio, second trial) nor the ISIS[3] (Second International Study of Infarct Survival) trials have demonstrated improved mortality associated with the use of rt-PA compared with streptokinase. Subsequent to the publication of the fourth edition of Brunwald (1992), the GUSTO (Global Utilization of Streptokinase and Tissue Plasminogen Activator for Occluded Coronary Arteries) trial revealed benefit of rt-PA vs. streptokinase in patients <75 years old with anterior myocardial infarction and in those presenting within 4 h of onset. See: Julian D & Brunwald E (1994) *Management of Acute Myocardial Infarction*. Saunders, London.
• The benefit of thrombolytic treatment is greatest when administered as early as possible after the onset of symptoms. Clear benefit is demonstrable when administered within 6 h and more so within 2 h.
• Benefit is only seen in the case of larger infarcts.
• Reduced rates of ventricular fibrillation, asystole and cardiogenic shock can be demonstrated in patients treated with thrombolytics (versus controls).
• Addition of aspirin to streptokinase treatment has been shown to have an additive effect. Heparin appears to prevent re-thrombosis, particularly after rt-PA use.
• The rate of intracerebral haemorrhage associated with thrombolytic use appears to be about 0.5%.

BRAUNWALD (1992) p. 1230

71. Systemic sclerosis
ANSWERS: c d

NOTES

• Systemic sclerosis is three to four times more common in females. Raynaud's phenomenon is a very common feature (70%). Those who never develop Raynaud's are more likely to be male and to have a high incidence of renal and myocardial involvement with a poor prognosis.

• There is oedema of the skin, especially of the fingers, progressing to fibrosis and calcinosis. Recurrent ulceration and secondary infection occur, especially at the finger tips.

• Telangiectasia occurs, especially over the limbs (there is no central arteriole, in contrast to the 'spider' telangiectasia of liver disease).

• Arthritis is non-erosive. Osteolysis with phalangeal tuft erosion contributes to the tapered appearance of the fingers.

• Oesophageal involvement is commonly observed radiologically (84%), ranging from absent peristalsis to oesophageal dilatation and spasm. Pathologically there is oesophageal muscle fibrosis. A minority of patients with demonstrable oesophageal abnormality have symptoms of dysphagia.

• Involvement of the small bowel results in prolonged transit time and bacterial overgrowth with malabsorption. There is a recognized association between systemic sclerosis and primary biliary cirrhosis.

• Alveolar thickening with reduced gas transfer is commonly found, with a restrictive pattern on lung function testing.

• Renal involvement (characterized by intimal proliferation and medial fibrinoid necrosis) with accelerated hypertension carries a poor prognosis since renal failure develops rapidly. Signs of micro-angiopathy, including fragmented red cells, are associated. Raised renin levels are associated but also occur commonly in patients not developing renal failure so can not be used to identify patients at risk.

• ANF is present in over 90% of cases but double standard (ds)-DNA binding is negative or positive in low titre. Rheumatoid factor is found in 30%. Anticentromere antibody is associated with limited systemic sclerosis and indicates a better prognosis.

• There are variants of systemic sclerosis which are thought to have a more favourable prognosis:

(a) localized; isolated skin and oesophageal involvement: progression to systemic disease is rare

(b) mixed connective tissue disease; antibody present to extractable nuclear antigen, arthralgia/arthritis, swollen hands, Raynaud's, abnormal oesophageal motility, myositis

(c) CREST syndrome—calcinosis, Raynaud's, abnormal oesophageal motility, sclerodactyly, telangiectasia.

KELLEY *et al.* (1993) p. 1113

72. Acute intermittent porphyria
ANSWERS: b c

NOTES
• Acute intermittent porphyria (AIP) is a consequence of porphobilinogen (PBG) deaminase deficiency. Inheritance is autosomal dominant and affected individuals have 50% of normal PBG deaminase activity.
• 90% of affected individuals remain asymptomatic throughout their lives.
• AIP is characterized by excessive hepatic production of porphyrin precursors (aminolaevulinic acid (ALA) and PBG). There is excessive urinary ALA and PBG excretion in the urine both between and during attacks (much more during attacks). Faecal porphyrin excretion is usually normal or slightly increased. The underlying enzyme defect can be identified in cultured fibroblasts.
• Clinical disease is manifested more frequently in females, only rarely presenting before puberty. High carbohydrate intake often reduces the frequency of attacks. Acute attacks may be precipitated by drugs, infection or starvation. Most cases are not adversely affected by pregnancy.
• Photosensitivity is very unusual in this variety of porphyria.
• Features of acute attacks include:
(a) autonomic disturbance, with abdominal pain, vomiting, constipation, tachycardia and sweating
(b) peripheral neuropathy, predominantly motor, usually preceded by myalgias or cramps: a complete flaccid paralysis may occur with loss of reflexes
(c) bulbar palsy or cerebellar signs (occasionally)
(d) agitation, confusion, disorientation and hallucinations.
• Hyponatraemia (thought to be a result of inappropriate ADH secretion), hypovolaemia and hypomagnesaemia may occur during acute attacks.
• Since the lesion is predominantly an axonal degeneration, peripheral nerve conduction during attacks tends to be relatively normal.
• In variegate porphyria (VP) there is a marked increase in faecal porphyrin excretion (especially protoporphyrin). PBG is excreted in excess in the urine only during acute attacks in VP.

SCRIVER et al. (1989) p. 1337
WALTON (1993) p. 597

73. Giant-cell arteritis
ANSWERS: a b c e

NOTES

• Giant-cell arteritis is an allergic arteritis affecting large and medium-sized arteries. Patients are generally aged over 60 years (mean 70 years). Females are affected twice as commonly as men.

• The condition may present as polymyalgia rheumatica, cranial arteritis or a combination of the two.

• Features of polymyalgia rheumatica include weight loss, depression, low-grade fever, severe morning stiffness (predominantly of girdle muscles), with pain and tenderness of these muscles.

• Cranial arteritis may result in temporal artery tenderness (with weak or absent pulsation) and headache (66%), masseter claudication, blindness (due to posterior ciliary or central retinal artery occlusion). Less commonly, transient cerebral ischaemic episodes, cranial or peripheral neuropathies may occur.

• About 15% of patients with polymyalgia rheumatica (without associated signs of arteritis) have giant-cell arteritis identified on temporal artery biopsy.

• The ESR is much raised in most cases. Temporal artery biopsy is positive in most cases of cranial arteritis (showing a granulomatous arteritis with giant cells). The lesions are discontinuous and biopsy of segments of artery which appear clinically abnormal gives a higher percentage of positive biopsies.

• Treatment is by corticosteroids; the dose is governed by the ESR response. The temporal artery biopsy remains positive for up to 40 h after the initiation of steroid therapy.

• The condition is self-limiting and treatment can be stopped in most patients, usually within 2 years.

KELLEY *et al.* (1993) p. 1103

74. Drug therapy in patients with AIP
ANSWERS: a d e

NOTES

• Drugs implicated as precipitants of acute porphyric attacks include barbiturates, carbamazepine, phenytoin, sodium valproate, sulphonamides, griseofulvin and ergot preparations.

• Drugs generally considered safe include narcotic analgesics, chloral hydrate, phenothiazines, penicillins, tetracyclines, streptomycin, corticosteroids, aspirin, paracetamol, atropine and suxamethonium.

SCRIVER *et al.* (1989) p. 1327

75. Bartter's syndrome
ANSWERS: a c d

NOTES
• Features of Bartter's syndrome include hypokalaemic alkalosis, with muscle cramps, polyuria, anorexia. The is increased aldosterone and elevated plasma renin activity.
• There is resistance to the effect of infused angiotensin and decreased responsiveness to noradrenaline.
• The juxtaglomerular apparatus is hypertrophied.
• Patients are characteristically normotensive, but orthostatic hypotension is a prominent fature.
• The primary abnormality appears to be a renal sodium and potassium loss, which may complicate a variety of tubular disorders.

DEGROOT (1995) pp. 1703, 2936

76. Diabetic nephropathy
ANSWERS: d e

NOTES
• In early, untreated juvenile diabetics both renal size and glomerular filtration rate are increased (30–40% above expected levels), possibly as a result of associated high growth hormone levels. The maximal capacity of the tubules to reabsorb glucose (TmG) is also increased.
• Expansion of the glomerular mesangial matrix and thickening of the basement membrane are early changes seen 18–36 months after the onset of IDDM. Kidneys are characteristically increased in size.
• In the early stages exercise-induced microalbuminaemia may be the only evidence of renal involvement.
• Microalbuminaemia is a sign of renal injury and greater than 30 mg/day is considered abnormal. Some 25–40% of patients with

IDDM have constant microalbuminaemia after 5–15 years.
• As renal disease progresses proteinuria increases (macroproteinuria >200 mg/day) and may cause nephrotic syndrome. Glomerular filtration rate (GFR) falls and hypertension is common.
• Almost all patients with established diabetic nephropathy have associated retinopathy.
• Red-cell casts are a feature of glomerulonephritis and are not characteristic of diabetic nephropathy.

DEGROOT (1995) p. 1569

77. Philadelphia chromosome
ANSWERS: d e

NOTES
• The Philadelphia chromosome (resulting from an unbalanced translocation of chromosomes 9 and 22 with partial deletion of a long arm of chromosome 22) is found in 95% of cases of CML, 20% of adults with acute lymphoblastic leukaemia (5% of children with acute lymphoblastic leukaemia or ALL) and 3% of cases of AML.
• The prognosis of ALL is worse in cases with Philadelphia chromosome.
• There have been a few reports of the Philadelphia chromosome in myelofibrosis, myeloid metaplasia and PRV. Such associations are very uncommon and some cases had had radiotherapy, known to predispose to CML.
• The abnormal chromosome occurs only in the myeloid, megakaryocyte and erythroid cell lines, not in lymphocytes or other cells.
• The abnormality persists during remission. Further chromosomal abnormalities are commonly seen when blast crisis supervenes.
• Atypical cases of chronic myeloid leukaemia (aCML) where the Philadelphia chromosome is not present (and there is no M-bcr rearrangement at a molecular level) have a worse prognosis than those cases where it is present (these cases are usually older and male). Mutated ras genes are rare in typical Philadelphia chromosome present (Ph +) CML but occur in >50% of cases of aCML.

LEE et al. (1993) pp. 1770, 1969, 2029

78. Urinary sediment
ANSWERS: b c e

NOTES
- Normal urinary protein loss is <100 mg/day, of which the predominant constituent is Tamm–Horsfall protein. Hyaline casts occur when there is low urine flow (e.g. where there is dehydration) due to gelling of this protein: they do not indicate renal disease.
- Small numbers of hyaline casts are normal and become much more frequent with fever or exercise, or following a dose of diuretic.
- Large numbers of broad hyaline casts suggest advanced chronic renal disease.
- Epithelial cells are a normal constituent of the urinary sediment. Epithelial-cell casts and coarse granular casts occur in acute tubular necrosis.
- White-cell casts are seen in pyelonephritis and occasionally in glomerulonephritis.
- Red cells will lyse in urine with a specific gravity below 1.006 (the morning sample has higher specific gravity so there is less chance of cell lysis). Glomerular red cells are characteristically of varying shape and haemoglobin content.
- Red-cell casts are indicative of glomerular damage.

SCHRIER & GOTTSCHALK (1993). p. 359

79. Variegate porphyria
ANSWERS: a b c d e

NOTES
- VP is inherited as an autosomal dominant—it is the predominant form of porphyria seen in South Africa (3/1000 whites).
- VP is caused by a deficiency of protoporphinogen oxidase activity.
- There is excessive PBG excretion in the urine only during attacks. Urinary coproporphyrin excretion usually exceeds uroporphyrin, except during attacks.
- There is usually a marked increase in faecal porphyrin excretion (which is not characteristic of AIP).
- Features are similar to those of AIP with the addition of photosensitivity. Of affected patients 33% only ever have cutaneous features and 15% never have skin lesions.

• The skin is abnormally fragile; on exposure to sunlight bullae develop. Healing occurs with scarring and pigmentation. Hypertrichosis is associated.
• As is the case with AIP, a high carbohydrate intake tends to reduce porphyrin production.

SCRIVER *et al.* (1989) p. 1341

80. Carcinoid syndrome
ANSWERS: c e

NOTES
• 95% of all carcinoids are found in the appendix, rectum and small intestine (about 1 : 300 appendices removed at appendicectomy contain carcinoids). Most of those arising elsewhere are sited in the bronchus.
• Small carcinoids <1 cm almost never metastasize, while those >2 cm almost always do.
• The carcinoid syndrome occurs in about 10% of cases with tumour and rarely, if ever, in hindgut tumours.
• Features include cutaneous flushing, sweating, venous telangiectasia, diarrhoea, bronchial constriction and abdominal pain. Cardiac vascular lesions, predominantly right-sided, occur later. Paroxysmal hypertension is not a feature.
• Flushing may be provoked by cheese, alcohol, β-adrenergic agonists, emotion and straining at stool. Attacks are generally transient, lasting for <5 min.
• Tryptophan is diverted from niacin production and pellagra may occur if the diet is deficient.
• Measurement of serotonin and its metabolites permits the detection of 84% of cases of neuroendocrine tumours. Ingestion of foods containing large quantities of serotonin interferes with interpretation of the results (e.g. bananas, pineapple, tomatoes, walnuts). In patients with foregut carcinoids the urine contains relatively little 5-hydroxyindoleacetic acid but large amounts of 5-hydroxytryptophan.
• Chromogranin A and B have been found to be elevated in all carcinoid patients.
• Hypokalaemia, hypercalcaemia and metabolic acidosis suggest vasoactive intestinal polypeptide (VIP)-secreting tumour rather than carcinoid.

DEGROOT (1995) p. 2803

81. Tetralogy of Fallot
ANSWER: b

NOTES

• Tetralogy of Fallot accounts for nearly 10% of cases of congenital heart disease. Associated cardiac anomalies are present in about 40% and extracardiac anomalies in 20%.

• In tetralogy of Fallot cyanosis occurs, or is intensified, as a result of (even mild) exercise. Most cases are cyanosed from birth and almost all become cyanosed by the end of the first year of life (it is the commonest cardiac malformation causing cyanosis after 1 year of age). Clubbing is prominent after 1 year.

• There is dyspnoea of effort; squatting reduces dysnoea and is employed by children with tetralogy of Fallot.

• Hypoxic attacks and syncope are serious complications (they are the commonest mode of death in this disease during infancy and childhood); they may be precipitated by infection, exertion, excitement and possibly by positively inotropic drugs.

• Angina on effort is extremely rare even in the presence of severe cyanosis.

• A pulmonary ejection murmur is frequently present, but not that of the ventricular septal defect which is usually large. The murmur may disappear during syncopal or cyanotic attacks.

• The second sound is nearly always single (since low pulmonary arterial pressure causes the pulmonary second sound to be very faint).

• There is right axis deviation and evidence of moderate right ventricular hypertrophy on the ECG. Right bundle branch block is not associated with tetralogy of Fallot.

• A right-sided aorta occurs in 25% of cases of tetralogy of Fallot. A boot-shaped heart (*coeur en sabot*) is characteristic on the chest X-ray.

BRAUNWALD (1992) p. 935

82. Bone marrow transplantation
ANSWERS: a c

NOTES

• Allogeneic or syngeneic bone marrow transplantation is capable of producing long-term disease-free survival in CML. Some 20% of those transplanted in blast crisis and 65% of those transplanted in chronic phase achieve a 5-year survival.

• Approximately 25% of patients with chronic disease will transform to acute-phase disease each year.

• Related donors with only one HLA A, B or D locus mismatch have a similar survival, as do HLA-identical sibling transplants. Mismatch at two or more loci is associated with increased graft rejection and GvHD.

• The lowest rate of relapse occurs in patients with acute and chronic GvHD. T-cell depletion from donor bone marrow reduces the risk of GvHD but is associated with increased risk of graft failure and an increased rate of leukaemia relapse.

• 20–50% of patients receiving marrow transplants from HLA-identical siblings develop significant acute GvHD.

• Cyclosporin reduces the rate of GvHD. Chronic GvHD usually responds to prednisolone (with or without cyclosporin) and in about 50% treatment can be discontinued within 1 year.

• Immunosuppression with increased liability to infection is a feature of both acute and chronic GvHD.

DEVITA, HELLMAN & ROSENBERG (1993) p. 1975
LEE *et al.* (1993) p. 701

83. Cushing's syndrome due to ectopic ACTH
ANSWERS: b c

NOTES
• Intrathoracic neoplasm (carcinoma of the bronchus, carcinoid of the bronchus or thymus) accounts for 60% of ectopic ACTH secretion. Other causes include pancreatic tumours, phaeochromocytoma and medullary carcinoma of the thyroid.

• Ectopic ACTH secretion occurs in 2% of all cases of lung cancer and 8% of those with small-cell tumours.

• In the ectopic ACTH syndrome the classic features of Cushing's syndrome are usually absent (central obesity, moon facies, striae and plethora).

• The very high levels of ACTH often seen in the ectopic syndrome may lead to skin pigmentation.

• Electrolyte imbalance, especially hypokalaemia alkalosis, may be associated with muscle weakness. Pulmonary and peripheral oedema are often prominent in the ectopic ACTH syndrome. Weight loss makes an ectopic aetiology more probable.

• In general there is more suppression of cortisol secretion in response to dexamethasone administration and more response to stimulation with CRH in Cushing's disease (pituitary hypersecretion of ACTH), than is the case with the ectopic ACTH syndrome.

• ACTH levels are within the normal range or moderately raised in Cushing's disease of pituitary origin but are characteristically very high in the ectopic syndrome.

• Of patients with ACTH-dependent Cushing's syndrome, about four times as many have Cushing's disease as have ectopic ACTH secretion.

DEGROOT *et al.* (1995) p. 1747

84. Psoriasis
ANSWERS: b d e

NOTES
• Psoriasis is common in Caucasians (1–2% of the population), but uncommon in those of Chinese origin. Psoriasis appears to be rare in the tropics.

• A familial history is obtainable in about 36% of cases.

• There are well-defined erythematous patches which bear large silvery scales. The extensor surfaces are especially affected; the face is usually spared (although the scalp is involved).

• Psoriasis exhibits the Kobner phenomenon. Itching is seldom a feature. Pitting, ridging and onycholysis of the nails is associated.

• Most cases are improved by sunlight, but photosensitivity may occur (about 5%), mainly in older female patients.

• Hyperuricaemia is associated—a reflection of the increased cell turnover.

• Treatment with local application of tar extract, dithranol or steroids may be effective. PUVA (a combination of psoralen administration and ultraviolet A irradiation) is beneficial. Methotrexate may be useful when the disease is severe.

• Antimalarials, β-blocking drugs and lithium are the drugs most frequently associated with exacerbation of psoriasis.

• The guttate variety is the type of psoriasis more commonly seen in children, often following streptococcal infection. This type has less tendency to chronicity than other varieties.

CHAMPION *et al.* (1992) p. 1391

85. Lichen planus
ANSWERS: b c d e

NOTES
• Lichen planus is characterized by papular skin lesions, usually small with a violaceous hue and with Wickham's striae on other surfaces. Itching is of variable severity. The hyperkeratotic variety (usually occurring on the ankles) and generalized types may itch severely.
• The mucous membranes are commonly involved (30–70%) and nails occasionally (10%). The genitals are frequently involved. The scalp is rarely affected but cicatricial alopecia results when it is involved. Residual pigmentation after lesions resolve may be intense.
• In 85% of cases lesions have cleared within 18 months. Mucosal lesions tend to persist longer than skin lesions.
• Drug-induced lichenoid eruption has been reported with gold, organic arsenicals, mepacrine, chloroquine, salicylate, streptomycin, tolbutamide, chlorpropamide and methyldopa.

CHAMPION et al. (1992) p. 1675

86. Dermatological manifestations of internal malignancy
ANSWERS: c d e

NOTES
• Acanthosis nigricans developing in adult life, in the absence of obesity, endocrine disturbance, excess nicotine acid ingestion or family history, is associated with an internal neoplasm in almost all cases (of the gastrointestinal tract in 90% of cases).
• Dermatomyositis, when it occurs in adults, is associated with neoplasia in up to 50% of cases.
• Erythema gyratum repens is a rare skin manifestation characterized by mobile, concentric, erythematous bands. It is usually associated with an internal neoplasm.
• Necrolytic migratory erythema appears to be specifically associated with a glucagon-secreting α islet cell tumour of the pancreas.
• Acquired ichthyosis occasionally occurs in association with lympho-reticular malignancies.
• The relationship between bullous pemphigoid and malignant disease remains controversial. However studies involving large numbers

of patients have not demonstrated an increased incidence of malignancies in patients with pemphigoid.

• Neither granuloma annulare nor necrobiosis lipoidica is associated with neoplasia.

CHAMPION *et al.* (1992) p. 2417

87. Leprosy
ANSWER: d

NOTES
• In tuberculois leprosy the disease remains predominantly neural. The plaque is the typical skin lesion: it is erythematous, hairless and anaesthetic. Nerve involvement may result in thickening and a localized, asymmetrical neuropathy.

• The skin smear is negative. Cell-mediated immunity is preserved and the lepromin test is strongly positive. IgM levels are normal.

• In lepromatous leprosy the skin lesions contain enormous numbers of bacilli, which may be seen on the skin smear. Skin lesions include macules, papules and nodules; they are not anaesthetic. Progression of the facial lesions may result in the classical leonine facies. Nasal involvement is common and causes stiffness and epistaxis.

• Cell-mediated immunity is depressed and the lepromin test is negative. IgM levels are increased. A biological false-positive test for syphilis, a positive titre of ANF and rheumatoid factor may be associated.

• Slow fibrosis of peripheral nerves in lepromatous leprosy results in bilateral symmetrical 'glove-and-stocking' anaesthesia.

CHAMPION *et al.* (1992) p. 1065

88. Uricosuric drugs
ANSWERS: d e

NOTES
• There are specific separate transport systems for the secretion and reabsorption of organic anions (including uric acid).

• Probenecid, phenylbutazone and sulphinpyrazone inhibit urate reabsorption and are therefore uricosuric.

• The uricosuric action of probenecid is blocked by salicylate which is an organic anion.

• Uricosuric drugs increase urate excretion and may cause uric acid crystal deposition in the collecting ducts (especially if the urine is acidic) or the production of urate stones.

• Diuretic-induced volume depletion leads to enhanced tubular reabsorption of uric acid as well as a decreased filtered load. Pyrazinamide, ethacrynic acid and ethanol also reduce renal urate clearance.

• Allopurinol is a xanthine-oxidase inhibitor. It has no action on the renal tubule but reduces uric acid production and thus excretion. Hypoxanthine and xanthine excretion is increased.

KELLEY *et al.* (1993) pp. 822, 1314

89. Haemophilia A
ANSWERS: a c e

NOTES
• Haemophilia is a sex-linked autosomal recessive condition. An affected male will not transmit the gene to his sons, but all of his daughters will be carriers.

• In about one-third of cases there is no family history of the disorder, the case being a result of a new mutation.

• Antigenically reactive (as measured by radioimmunoassay) factor VIIIc is present in the plasma of most haemophiliacs.

• The partial thromboplastin time (PTT) is usually prolonged in patients with haemophilia A. The prothrombin time PT is normal.

• Antibodies to factor VIIIc can be identified in up to 20% of patients with haemophilia A.

• Polymorphic DNA probes are able to identify 96% of carriers.

LEE *et al.* (1993) p. 1424

90. Minimal-change nephrotic syndrome
ANSWER: a

NOTES
• MCNS accounts for 80% of cases of nephrotic syndrome occurring between the ages of 1 and 5 years; it is less common in other age groups but may be responsible for up to 20% of adult cases of nephrotic syndrome.

• Selective proteinuria is characteristic. IgG levels are reduced to about 20% of normal while IgM levels are increased.

• Microscopic haematuria occurs in 30% of cases, but is almost never macroscopic.

• Hypertension is an unusual association (<20%).

• Serum albumin concentrations of <20 g/l are usual in children with MCNS while levels of α_2-and β-globulins are increased.

• Mild transient uraemia is common.

• The serum C3 and C4 complement levels are almost invariably normal in MCNS.

• Electron microscopy of biopsy material shows fusion of the foot processes of the glomerular epithelial cells. The glomerular basement membrane appears normal and there is no deposition of immune complexes or complement.

• Corticosteroids greatly accelerate the tendency to slow spontaneous remission in the majority of cases (90% have protein-free urine by 4 weeks). Relapse occurs in about 25% of cases, frequently occurring several times. There is generally less tendency to relapse as time passes. Cyclophosphamide may induce long periods of remission in patients who relapse frequently.

SCHRIER & GOTTSCHALK (1993) p. 1731

91. Wolff–Parkinson–White syndrome
ANSWERS: a b c d e

NOTES

• In Wolff–Parkinson–White syndrome there is a short PR interval (<0.12 s) and a prolonged QRS interval (longer than 0.12 s).

• Positive QRS complexes have a slurred upstroke (the δ wave); those which are negative have a slurred downstroke preceding the QRS or QR. (A deep Q wave results in lead III).

• The T-wave changes are secondary to the QRS and thus when the QRS is strongly positive there is T-wave inversion (e.g. in leads I and aVL).

• The electrocardiographic pattern may completely obscure the changes of myocardial infarction.

• Frequency of attacks of tachycardia increases with age (10% cases <40 years, 36% cases >60 years). Wide QRS complexes do not occur during the tachycardia. Approximately 80% of cases have a reciprocating tachycardia, 15–30% have atrial fibrillation and 5% have flutter. Very rapid ventricular rates may complicate atrial fibrillation.

• A short PR interval, normal QRS interval, absent δ wave and bouts of tachycardia are features of the Lown–Ganong–Levine syndrome.

• Pre-excitation is more common in relatives of patients with Wolff–Parkinson–White syndrome than in the normal population.

• Drugs are used to increase the refractory period of the atrioventricular node, accessory pathway or both. Verapamil, propranolol, adenosine and digoxin all prolong the refractory period of atrioventricular node. Verapamil and propranolol do not incease the refractory period of the accessory pathway while digoxin may enhance accessory pathway conduction and is contraindicated as a sole agent. Class IA and IC drugs prolong the refractory period of the accessory pathway.

BRAUNWALD (1992) p. 693

92. Extensor plantar reflexes and absent knee jerks
ANSWERS: a b c d e

NOTES
• Spinal cord compression at the third and fourth lumbar levels results in a flaccid paralysis of quadriceps and hip abductor muscles with diminution or loss of the knee jerks. Upper motor neuron lesion signs occur below the fourth lumbar level with spastic paralysis, exaggerated ankle jerks and extensor plantar reflexes.

• In motor neuron disease there is degeneration of anterior horn cells and the corticospinal tracts. Reflexes may be exaggerated or absent (depending on the degree of corticospinal tract damage) and the plantar reflexes often become extensor.

• Corticospinal tract involvement commonly occurs in multiple sclerosis leading to hyperreflexia and extensor plantar reflexes. Occasionally severe sensory involvement may cause the reflex arc to be broken and reflexes to disappear.

• Reflexes are diminished in tabes dorsalis, but the plantar reflexes are flexor unless there is associated taboparesis and corticospinal tract damage.

• Subacute combined degeneration of the cord (which may complicate pernicious anaemia) is associated with peripheral neuropathy, corticospinal tract and posterior column damage. Loss of tendon reflexes and extensor plantar reflexes may be seen.

• Ataxia, nystagmus, posterior column and corticospinal tract degeneration (with extensor plantar reflexes) and loss of tendon reflexes are features of Friedreich's ataxia.

WALTON (1993) pp. 295, 366, 434, 443, 493, 537

93. Friedreich's ataxia
ANSWERS: a b c d e

NOTES
• Friedreich's ataxia is the commonest of the early-onset ataxias (50% of all hereditary ataxias). Inheritance is autosomal recessive.
• Pathologically there is degeneration of the posterior columns and spinocerebellar tract—most severe in the cervical region—and loss of dorsal root ganglia cells. The brainstem, cerebellum and cerebrum are relatively normal.
• First symptoms, usually gait ataxia, occur between the ages of 8 and 15 years with absent tendon reflexes. Rombergism is usually present at the time of diagnosis.
• Axonal sensory neuropathy is demonstrated on electrophysiology.
• Dysarthria, upper motor neuron weakness with extensor plantar reflexes, loss of joint position sense and vibration sense are eventually found in all cases.
• Visual evoked potentials are of reduced amplitude and somewhat delayed latency occurs in most cases.
• The ECG is abnormal in 65% of cases. Widespread T-wave inversion is common.
• 95% of cases are chairbound by the age of 45.
• The differential diagnosis includes hereditary motor and sensory neuropathy type 1 and abetalipoproteinaemia.

WALTON (1993) p. 432

94. Coeliac disease
ANSWERS: a c e

NOTES
• A family history of coeliac disease is obtained in many cases; there is an association with the histocompatibility antigen HLA-B8, which

occurs in 60–90% of coeliac patients but in only 20% of the general population.

• Gluten consumption results in the development of villous atrophy, which is most pronounced in the duodenum and proximal jejunum, decreasing in severity in the ileum. Crypt hyperplasia and inflammatory cell infiltration of the lamina propria are associated.

• Fat malabsorption leads to deficiency of fat-soluble vitamins. Hypocalcaemia is frequent, although Chvostek's or Trousseau's signs are rarely elicited; secondary hyperparathyroidism may result. There is protein malabsorption and excessive protein loss into the gut (protein-losing enteropathy).

• Interstitial mucosal disaccharidase deficiency is an almost invariable accompaniment of coeliac disease. The xylose tolerance test is abnormal (reduced levels of xylose in the urine). However, urinary xylose excretion is influenced by renal blood flow.

• Intestinal hypomobility is characteristic and small-bowel transit time increased. Jejunal dilatation is common.

• Skin pigmentation is common; clubbing and epidermal ridge atrophy are associated.

• There is an increased risk of lymphoma in patients with coeliac disease. Carcinoma of the oesophagus and small-bowel adenocarcinoma are both associated with coeliac disease.

• Gluten is a water-soluble protein constituent of wheat, barley and rye flour but is not present in rice or cornflour. Gluten content of oat flour is variable. Application of gluten to the mucosa of a susceptible patient results in a classic mucosal lesion and symptoms within 8–12 h.

SLEISENGER & FORDTRAN (1993) p. 1078

95. Cataract
ANSWERS: a c d e

NOTES
• Progressive clouding of the cornea is almost universal in Hurler's syndrome; it is rare in Hunter's syndrome.
• Subcapsular cataract complicates hypocalcaemia.
• Cataract is a feature of congenital rubella. Lens opacities occur in up to 75% of cases of Down's syndrome.

- In galactosaemia, cataracts often develop during childhood and may also develop in early adult life in heterozygotes (with mild disease expression).
- Cataract is a well-recognized complication of diabetes mellitus.
- Cataract commonly occurs in dystrophia myotonica and may be associated with atopic dermatitis.
- Still's disease (usually those cases with a positive test for ANF) may be complicated by iritis and cataract. Cataract does not appear to occur more frequently in patients with scleroderma than in the general population.
- Cerebrotendinous xanthomatosis is a rare recessive disorder characterized by cataracts, xanthomas, severe neurological deficiencies, dementia and cardiovascular disease. There is an elevated circulating cholestanol level in the plasma.

DEGROOT et al. (1995) pp. 1124, 2741
KELLEY et al. (1993) pp. 512, 514
SCRIVER et al. (1989) pp. 471, 1565

96. Liver disease and steroid therapy
ANSWERS: c d

NOTES
- Gilbert's syndrome (familial unconjugated non-haemolytic hyperbilirubinaemia) is characterized by a mild jaundice. This may be reduced by hepatic enzyme induction resulting from phenobarbitone therapy. Corticosteroids are ineffective.
- Corticosteroids are contraindicated in primary biliary cirrhosis. Although they reduce itching and result in a fall in alkaline phosphatase concentration, the increased osteoporosis which occurs is a serious problem and outweighs the advantage.
- Prednisolone improves both well-being and prognosis in chronic active hepatitis.
- Corticosteroids do not alter the degree of liver necrosis, accelerate the rate of healing or assist in immunity to virus hepatitis. They do however result in a rapid fall of serum bilirubin and transaminase levels are of diagnostic and therapeutic value where prolonged cholestasis follows viral hepatitis A.
- Steroids are not of established benefit in acute hepatic failure.

SHERLOCK & DOOLEY (1993) pp. 209, 236, 265, 304

97. Hyperkalaemia
ANSWER: e

NOTES
• In hyperkalaemia the P-wave amplitude is diminished and the PR interval may be increased, progressing to atrial standstill. Atrial fibrillation may occur. There is widening of the QRS complexes and diminished R-wave amplitude. The T waves become large and 'tented'. These changes are exaggerated by associated hyponatraemia.
• In hypokalaemia the P waves may become peaked and the PR interval increased. There is depression of the ST segment, the T waves become flattened and the U wave becomes more prominent.
• In hypocalcaemia the ST segment of the ECG is isoelectric but prolonged (result in a prolonged QT interval).

BRAUNWALD (1992) p. 149

98. Generalized pruritus
ANSWERS: a c e

NOTES
• Causes of generalized pruritis include:
(a) generalized skin disease (e.g. erythroderma, eczema, varicella and occasionally rubella)
(b) allergy to infestation (e.g. scabies, onchocerciasis)
(c) drug and food reactions
(d) cholestasis
(e) endocrine (myxoedema, thyrotoxicosis, hyperparathyroidism)
(f) chronic renal failure (possibly as a result of associated hyperparathyroidism)
(g) neoplasia (especially Hodgkin's disease and PRV)
(h) iron deficiency
(i) psychogenic disorders.
• The association of diabetes with generalized pruritis is under dispute.
• The cutaneous manifestations of secondary syphilis do not itch.

HART (1985) p. 689

99. Motor neuron disease
ANSWERS: a b c

NOTES
• In MND there is degeneration of anterior horn cells and corticospinal tracts of the spinal cord and of the motor nuclei in the brainstem (however the third, fourth and sixth nuclei are less affected than lower nuclei).
• The Betz cells of the motor cortex are depleted in patients with predominant upper motor neuron signs.
• There is weakness, wasting and fasciculation of involved muscles combined with signs of corticospinal tract damage (spasticity, hyperreflexia and extensor plantar reflexes).
• There is no sensory impairment, though there may be cramp-like pain in involved muscles in later stages.
• Pseudobulbar palsy (resulting from upper motor neuron damage) occurs and is associated with impaired voluntary control of emotional response; however, intellect is not impaired. When the medulla is involved there is usually evidence of both upper and lower motor neuron damage.
• Nerve conduction velocity is normal (except in the very late stages when demyelination may follow axonal degeneration)., The EMG shows fibrillation and fasciculation potentials.
• There may be a modest rise of serum enzymes reflecting muscle damage (e.g. creatinine phosphokinase).

WALTON (1993) p. 443

100. Urinary-reducing substances
ANSWERS: a b c d e

NOTES
• The Clinitest reaction becomes positive (changes from blue to orange) in the presence of a reducing agent; in clinical practice this is usually glucose.
• Other agents giving a positive reaction include lactose, pentose, fructose, galactose and homogentisic acid (excreted in alkaptonuria).
• Drugs associated with a positive reaction include salicylates, isoniazid, levodopa, ascorbic acid, nalidixic acid and tetracyclines.
• The enzymatic (glucose oxidase) test (Diastix) is specific for glucose.

The reaction may be inhibited by the presence of levodopa, ascorbic acid or ketones.

HART (1985) p. 310

101. Rheumatic fever
ANSWERS: a c

NOTES
• A limited number of streptococcal serotypes appear to be associated with acute rheumatic fever. Strains are characteristically mucoid (highly encapsulated).
• Nephritogenic group A streptococci rarely if ever cause acute rheumatic fever.
• Following pharyngitis caused by virulent rheumatogenic strains of streptococci, about 3% of those infected can be predicted to develop rheumatic fever.
• Rheumatic fever does not seem to occur after streptococcal skin infection.
• Reactivation following subsequent streptococcal infections is much more common in those who have previously suffered an attack of rheumatic fever.
• Features of rheumatic fever include arthritis (large-joint), carditis, chorea, subcutaneous nodules and erythema marginatum (these are the major diagnostic criteria).
• Rheumatic chorea is characterized by spontaneous movement, ataxia, weakness and hypotonia. Emotional expression may be impaired. It occurs predominantly in adolescent females (virtually never in adult men). Movements cease during sleep.
• A raised ASO titre is an indication of recent streptococcal infection but is not a measure of rheumatic activity. Titres fall during rheumatic fever unless there is intercurrent streptococcal infection.
• Young children with rheumatic fever have the highest insidence of carditis (>90%).

KELLEY et al. (1993) p. 1209

102. Osteogenesis imperfecta

ANSWERS: a e

NOTES

• OI is associated with abnormal type I collagen synthesis.

• OI can be classified into four types:

(a) type I: dominant inheritance, blue sclerae, normal teeth, near normal stature, variable number of long bone fractures (decreased production of type 1 procollagen)

(b) type II: severe perinatal lethal form with minimal calvarial calcification, compressed long bone fractures resulting from a heterogeneous range of genetic and biochemical disorders.

(c) type III: predominantly dominant inheritance, usually deformity at birth due to *in utero* fractures with more fractures subsequently. There is general osteopenia, marked shortening of stature and kyphoscoliosis. Dentinogenesis is common. There is variable scleral blueness which lightens with age.

(d) type IV: dominant inheritance, normal sclerae, dentinogenesis, mild-to-moderate bone deformity.

• In OI there is no increased risk of sarcoma development and cataracts are not a feature.

• Blue sclerae are characteristic, particularly of type I OI, but may also occur in Marfan's and Ehlers–Danlos syndromes.

• Hearing loss is a common feature beginning in the teens and becoming profound by the fourth or fifth decade.

SCRIVER *et al.* (1989) p. 2805

103. Psoriatic arthropathy

ANSWER: e

NOTES

• Psoriatic arthritis is often associated with severe skin disease; however it may precede the development of skin disease. Nail changes are frequently found in association with joint disease.

• Peripheral (especially interphalangeal) joints are mainly involved; involvement is less symmetrical than in rheumatoid arthritis. The very destructive mutilans type of disease is rare (5%).

• Sacroiliitis is common (10–30% of cases of arthritis), often associated with the HLA B27 tissue type. Conjunctivitis and iritis also occur.

• Conjunctivitis complicates about 20% while iritis occurs in about 7% (usually associated with sacroiliitis).
• >20 fingernail pits suggests psoriasis while more than 60 is only seen in psoriasis.
• A severe psoriasform rash and arthropathy is a recognized feature of AIDS.

KELLEY *et al.* (1993) p. 974

104. Short stature
ANSWERS: c d e

NOTES
• Pathological causes of short stature include:
(a) chromosomal abnormalities (e.g. Turner's syndrome, Down's syndrome)
(b) skeletal abnormalities (e.g. achondroplasia, Brailsford–Morquio's disease, Hurler's syndrome, OI, rickets)
(c) endocrine disorders (hypothyroidism, hypopituitarism and isolated growth hormone deficiency, PHP, precocious puberty)
(d) chronic childhood illness
(e) chronic renal failure, congenital heart disease, malabsorption, malnutrition, fibrocystic disease
(f) syndromes (Lawrence–Moon–Biedl, Fröhlich, DeLange, von Gierke's).
• Children with cirrhosis tend to be of normal height or taller than their peers. Patients with Marfan's syndrome and homocystinuria are also tall.

HART (1985) p. 798
SHERLOCK & DOOLEY (1993) p. 446

105. Hypoglycaemia
ANSWERS: a b d

NOTES
• In glycogenosis type I (von Gierke's disease) there is hepatic and renal glucose-6-phosphatase deficiency. There is a severe tendency to hypoglycaemia.
• Galactosaemia results from galactose-2-phosphate uridyl transferase

deficiency. Hypoglycaemia occurs on exposure to galactose in the diet.
• There is hypoglycaemia in hereditary fructose intolerance after ingestion of fructose or sucrose (note that neither occurs in breast milk).
• In glycogenosis type II (Pompe's disease) due to lysosomal acid maltase deficiency hypoglycaemia does not occur.
• Hypoglycaemia is not a feature of Gaucher's disease.
• G6PD deficiency is characterized by haemolysis. Hypoglycaemia is not a feature.

SCRIVER *et al.* (1989) pp. 407, 433, 471, 1678, 2789

106. Tay–Sachs disease
ANSWER: d

NOTES
• The gangliosidoses are autosomal recessive disorders.
• Tay–Sachs disease refers to the most severe infantile form of the disorder. It occurs in most races but is much more common among Ashkenazi Jews (100 times more frequent).
• Hexosaminidase deficiency is the molecular basis of Tay–Sachs disease and cerebral accumulation of GM2 ganglioside is pathognomonic.
• Affected babies are normal during the first postnatal months, but develop slowly and fall behind developmental milestones. Retardation is usually quite obvious by 8 months.
• The child's activity decreases and it is easily startled. Fits may occur and eventually cortical blindness ensues. Increased head circumference is characteristic (approximately 50% greater than normal by 2 years of age).
• The cherry-red spot develops in the macular region within the first year (this also occurs in 30% of cases of Niemann–Pick disease).
• There is no organomegaly or overt involvement of the bony skeleton.
• Syringomyelin accumulation occurs in Niemann–Pick disease.

SCRIVER *et al.* (1989) p. 1829

107. Felty's syndrome
ANSWER: c

NOTES
• About two-thirds of patients with Felty's syndrome are female.

• HLA-DRw4 is found in 95% of patients with Felty's syndrome, 70–75% of patients with rheumatoid arthritis and 30–35% of normal controls.

• Felty's syndrome is generally associated with severe erosive rheumatoid joint disease of >10 years' duration.

• There is granulocytopenia and splenomegaly. The degree of splenomegaly is unrelated to the severity of granulocytopenia. Liability to bacterial infection is increased.

• Abnormal liver function occurs in about 25% of cases.

• Rheumatoid factor is characteristically positive in high titre and ANF is present in 66% of cases with antihistone antibodies (SSA, SSB) often in high titre.

• Immunoglobulin levels are generally higher than in patients with rheumatoid arthritis but no Felty's syndrome.

• Increased splenic sequestration and removal of granulocytes have been demonstrated in Felty's syndrome. Splenectomy results in increased granulocyte counts within minutes to hours in 88% of cases.

• In most cases marrow examination shows myeloid hyperplasia with a relative excess of immature forms (maturation arrest). Demonstration of *in vitro* inhibition of humoral colony stimulation by serum from patients with Felty's syndrome suggests that this may be an additional factor contributing to granulocytopenia.

• Spontaneous remissions are uncommon.

KELLEY *et al.* (1993) p. 924

108. Interferon

ANSWERS: b c d e

NOTES

• IFN-α is synthesized predominantly by lymphocytes and monocytes while β-interferon (IFN-β) is secreted by fibroblasts. IFN-γ is produced by T cells and natural killer (NK) cells.

• Viruses are the most effective inducers of interferons (RNA viruses are more effective stimulators of interferons than are DNA viruses). Administration of antibodies to interferons results in more severe viral infections in animals.

• Interferons bind to specific cell receptors with a common receptor for IFN-α and IFN-β, with a second receptor for IFN-γ

• IFN-γ is a major activator of macrophages.

- Rigors, fever, myalgia and anorexia occur with therapeutic administration of recombinant interferons.
- IFN-α has been shown to be effective in chronic hepatitis C.

LACHMANN *et al.* (1993) pp. 315, 1502, 1818

109. Insulinoma
ANSWERS: a b c e

NOTES
- 6% of insulinomas are malignant. The remainder are adenomas, 9% of which are multiple, and half of whom have the MEN I syndrome.
- Few patients with insulinoma are aged less than 20 years; median age at diagnosis is about 50 years (except in those with the MEN I syndrome, when the median onset is mid 20s).
- 60% of cases of insulinoma occur in women.
- In those with the MEN I syndrome 60% have multiple tumours. Hyperparathyroidism is the commonest associated endocrine abnormality.
- Insulinomas have not been detected in insulin-dependent diabetics.
- There is characteristically hypoglycaemia after fasting and exercise with inappropriately high insulin levels (92% of cases become hypoglycaemic if fasted for 48 h). Stimulation of insulin release, to aid diagnosis, may be achieved by administration of tolbutamide. Leucine or glucagon stimulates insulin release but glycine does not.
- 80% of patients with insulinoma have raised proinsulin concentrations (>20% of total immunoreactive insulin).
- Hypoglycaemia may complicate large tumours, especially for mesenchymal origin (fibromas, sarcomas), or hepatomas. The hypoglycaemia may be a result of tumour secretion of an insulin-like substance or excessive glucose utilization by the tumour.

DEGROOT *et al.* (1995) p. 1612

110. Interleukins
ANSWERS: b c d e

NOTES
- Interleukin 1 (IL-1) is secreted in response to infection and inflammation. It stimulates T cells, C-reactive protein synthesis,

pituitary ACTH release and is an endogenous pyrogen.

• IL-1 stimulates tumour necrosis factor and IL-6 release, but IL-6 does not stimulate IL-1 release.

• Activation of T cells causes release of IL-2. Receptors for IL-2 are not present on resting (unstimulated) T cells but are present 24 h after activation. IL-2 interaction with receptors results in non-specific T-cell proliferation.

• IL-4, IL-5 and IL-6 mediate T-cell stimulation of B-cell proliferation and antibody secretion.

LACHMANN *et al.* (1993) pp. 267, 287, 299

111. Herpes zoster
ANSWERS: b c d

NOTES

• Herpes zoster usually occurs in older adults but can occur in children. Patients with herpes zoster may give varicella (chickenpox) to exposed susceptible individuals.

• The eruption, usually limited to one or two adjacent dermatomes, most frequently occurs over the thoracic and lumbar dermatomes. A few vesicles in other areas than the main affected dermatomes are not uncommon. Severe generalized infection may occur, usually under conditions of immunosuppression.

• Involvement of the maxillary and mandibular branches of the trigeminal nerve is much less common than is involvement of the ophthalmic branch.

• Pain usually precedes the rash. Erythema precedes the development of vesicles.

• Tender local lymphadenopathy is common in the early stages of the rash.

• Persistent neuralgic pain continues in 25–50% of cases, especially in older patients. Secondary infection is frequent (particularly dangerous in ophthalmic infection). Meningoencephalitis is a rare complication; recovery is usual.

• Motor nerves may be involved and motor paralysis ensue (lower motor neuron type), as in the Ramsay Hunt syndrome (pain and vesicles in the external auditory meatus, loss of taste in the anterior two-thirds of the tongue and ipsilateral facial palsy).

• Acyclovir results in more rapid healing, prevention of the development of new lesions and a reduced period of viral isolation from lesions if begun early after onset. Reduction of pain or postherpetic neuralgia remains unproven.

MANDELL, BENNETT & DOLIN (1995) p. 1153

112. Pertussis
ANSWER: all incorrect

NOTES
• Pertussus is highly infectious. Infants are very susceptible and most deaths occur in those infected in the first year of life. Females are more succeptible than males. Maternal antibody does not appear to confer significant protection from this infection.
• Vaccination does not confer lifelong immunity and adults may become infected (10% of reported cases are more than 15 years old) and transmit the infection to young children.
• There is a catarrhal stage lasting about 1 week followed by a spasmodic stage with paroxysms of coughing leading to cyanosis and sometimes followed by vomiting.
• Pertussis is associated with a lymphocytosis.
• Complications include subconjuctival haemorrhage (secondary to coughing); convulsions (2% more common and persistent than with other infections); coma (this has a poor prognosis and hemiplegia may persist in survivors). Lung collapse is the commonest respiratory complication; secondary bronchopneumonia is a serious development.
• Antibiotic treatment early during the first week of infection may attenuate the disease. Erythromycin may reduce the period of infectivity.

MANDELL, BENNETT & DOLIN (1995) p. 1757

113. Intracerebral calcification
ANSWERS: a c d e

NOTES
• Glioblastoma multiforme is a rapidly growing cerebral tumour. Calcification does not develop. The slow-growing oligodendroglioma may become calcified. Craniopharyngiomas are frequently calcified;

140

angiomas and meningiomas occasionally calcify.

• Fine curvilinear calcification can occur in aneurysms. Widespread calcification outlining gyri of a parietal and/or occipital lobe is seen in Sturge–Weber syndrome.

• Multiple flakes of subcortical calcification are characteristic of congenital toxoplasmosis; in addition there may be basal ganglia calcification. (Other features include spasticity, mental deficiency and choroidoretinitis.)

• In cysticercosis, cysts may occur in muscle and brain. The cysts become calcified in time (usually after about 10 years). Muscle cysts calcify before those in the brain. Epilepsy commonly complicates cerebral involvement.

• Tuberculomas and chronic intracerebral haematomas may develop areas of calcification.

• Patchy intracerebral calcification may develop in tuberose sclerosis (features of this condition include cerebral gliosis, adenoma sebaceum (this only develops after 5 years of age) hamartomatous tumours, bone cysts, epilepsy and mental subnormality). Note that there is a predisposition to glioma development in tuberose sclerosis.

• Calcification of the basal ganglia occurs in PHP and hypoparathyroidism. Minor calcification is also common in elderly patients and is a feature of lead intoxication.

WALTON (1993) pp. 160, 311, 313, 404, 466

114. PR interval
ANSWERS: a c e

NOTES

• The normal PR interval is between 0.12 and 0.21 s; there is a trend toward the longer period with age. The PR interval becomes shorter at more rapid rates (except at very rapid rates, when the refractory period of the atrioventricular node is infringed upon).

• An abnormally short PR interval occurs in the Wolff–Parkinson–White syndrome (short PR, prolonged QRS duration and δ waves with bouts of tachycardia) and Lown–Ganong–Levine syndrome (short PR interval but normal QRS complexes and bouts of tachycardia).

• The PR interval is also commonly short in Duchenne muscular dystrophy, type II glycogen storage disease (Pompe's disease) and in HOCM.

• A long PR interval constitutes first-degree heart block. First-degree heart block is common in atrial septal defect, cardiomyopathy, rheumatic carditis, SBE and dystrophia myotonica and may occur in ischaemic heart disease. Digoxin, procainamide and quinidine therapy may be associated with first-degree heart block. Lignocaine and phenytoin either have no significant effect on the atrioventricular node or accelerate conduction (i.e. are associated with a short PR interval).

BRAUNWALD (1992) pp. 120, 135, 1404, 1645, 1811

115. Niacin deficiency
ANSWERS: a b c d

NOTES
• Niacin (nictonic acid, nicotinamide, vitamin B_2) deficiency results in the development of pellagra. Nicotinic acid may be produced by metabolism of the essential amino acid tryptophan in the body.
• Nicotine acid is metabolized to nicotinamide adenine dinucleotide (NAD) and nicotinamide adenine dinucleotide phosphate (NADP): these are important reducing agents.
• Features of pellagra include a characteristic photosensitive dermatitis, dementia (usually preceded by a depression) and glossitis.
• Neurological damage associated with niacin deficiency includes cerebral oedema and atrophy, long tract (spinal cord) and peripheral demyelination. The neurological signs may resemble those seen in subacute combined degeneration of the cord.
• Pellagra may complicate alcoholism, malabsorption and Hartnup disease (an inborn error of metabolism in which there is cerebellar ataxia, aminoaciduria and excess urinary indoleacetic acid excretion). Isoniazid therapy is occasionally complicated by pellagra (isoniazid is a pyridoxine antagonist; this agent is essential for the convertion of tryptophan to nicotinic acid).
• If there is low dietary niacin intake then pellagra may develop in carcinoid syndrome (since tryptophan is utilized in the excessive 5-hydroxytryptamine synthesis).
• There is a reduced urinary excretion of N'-methylnicotinamide in pellagra. However, the clinical features and response to therapy usually establish the diagnosis.
• Treatment is with nicotinamide; however, the deficiency is usually

multiple and thiamine and riboflavine are usually administered in addition.

WALTON (1993) p. 534

116. Hurler's syndrome
ANSWERS: b d e

NOTES
• Hurler's syndrome is a mucopolysaccharidosis (designated type I) which results from α-L-iduronidase deficiency.
• Features of the syndrome include dwarfism, kyphosis, short extremities, stiff joints with contractures, scaphocephaly, grotesque facies (hence the alternative name gargoylism) including hypertelorism and enlarged tongue and lips. Cataracts, conductive nerve deafness, hepatosplenomegaly, cardiomyopathy and cardiac valvular damage also occur.
• Severe mental retardation occurs; this is usually evident by the end of the first year of life.
• In Hurler's syndrome death usually occurs before the age of 10.
• All of the mucopolysaccharidoses are inherited as autosomal recessives, except Hunter's, which is an X-linked disorder.
• Mental retardation is absent or slight in Morquio's syndrome (type IV), Scheie syndrome and type VI mucopolysaccharidosis.
• Prenatal diagnosis can be made by examining chorionic villus biopsies for enzyme activity.

SCRIVER et al. (1989) p. 1571

117. Hepatocellular liver disease
ANSWERS: c d

NOTES
• Clotting factors I, II, V, VII, IX and X are produced by the liver. Factor VII is the earliest to be reduced in liver disease, followed by factors II and X. Factor I and V levels persist in the face of severe liver disease better than levels of the other factors.
• Factor VIII is not produced by the liver and levels are uninfluenced by liver disease.
• Factors II, VII, IX and X are well-preserved in banked blood. Factor

143

V is only present in significant quantities in fresh blood; however, this factor is usually well-preserved in liver disease and the bleeding diathesis of liver disease may be effectively reversed by infusion of banked blood.

• Hepatocellular disease and cholestasis are associated with the development of target cells. Spur cells are a late feature and are associated with far-advanced liver disease.

• Percutaneous liver biopsy is contraindicated if the PT is prolonged for >3 s beyond that of the control.

• In both acute and chronic liver disease there is an increased plasma concentration of aromatic amino acids (tyrosine, phenylalanine and methionine), while the levels of branched-chain amino acids (leucine, isoleucine and valine) are reduced.

SHERLOCK & DOOLEY (1993) p. 72

118. Infectious mononucleosis
ANSWERS: a e

NOTES

• In developed countries infectious mononucleosis has a maximum incidence among adolescents and young adults. Children become infected, especially under conditions of overcrowding (50% of children seroconvert before the age of 5). In children infection is frequently subclinical.

• Clinical infection is usually characterized by lymphadenopathy (94%) and fever (76%). Splenomegaly occurs in about 50%, but hepatomegaly is less common (12%).

• Hepatitis occurs in most cases and abnormal liver function tests are usual (>80%). Jaundice is uncommon. Thrombocytopenia or autoimmune haemolytic anaemia (3% of cases due to an IgM cold agglutinin) are recognized complications. Neurological complications are rarely associated. Splenic rupture is a risk in infectious mononucleosis. Upper airway obstruction is a recognized complication.

• Atypical mononucleated cells are associated with infectious mononucleosis; they constitute about 30% of the total white-cell count. In most cases there is a leukocytosis of between 10 000 and 20 000 cells/m^3. Atypical mononuclear cells may also occur in CMV, toxoplasmosis, rubella, hepatitis and some drug reactions, but generally not in such numbers as in infectious mononucleosis.

144

• Heterophile antibody (agglutinin) is found in the serum of 90% of patients with infectious mononucleosis. It is the basis of the Paul–Bunnell test. The heterophile antibody agglutinates sheep red blood cells. It is absorbed by ox red cells but not guinea-pig kidney.

• 90–95% of adults have antibodies to Epstein–Barr virus. Epstein–Barr virus can be isolated from throat washings of up to 20% of normal healthy adults.

• The development of a maculopapular rash after administration of ampicillin to patients with infectious mononucleosis is extremely common. The rash is distinct from that associated with hypersensitivity to all penicillins.

MANDELL, BENNETT & DOLIN (1995) p. 1172

119. Mendelian X-linked dominant conditions
ANSWERS: a d e

NOTES

• A Mendelian X-linked condition can affect, and be transmitted by, both males and females.

• Affected females may be either heterozygous or homozygous for the mutant gene. If the disease is expressed in the female heterozygote it is refered to as X-linked dominant and if only in the female homozygote, then X-linked recessive. All males will express the full disease since they carry only one X chromosome.

• Affected females transmit the condition to half of their children, whether male or female.

• Affected males pass the defective X chromosome to all of their daughters, but to none of their sons (since no X chromosome is transmitted to them from their father).

• An X-linked dominant disorder should be observed in females twice as often as in males.

• The classical example of an X-linked dominantly inherited condition is familial hypophosphataemic rickets.

SCRIVER et al. (1989) p. 26

120. Cutaneous anthrax

ANSWER: c

NOTES

• *Bacillus anthracis* is a Gram-positive spore-forming rod. Serological diagnosis is possible using a haemagglutination test.
• Humans are very resistant to infection. Those working with animal hides and fleeces are inevitably exposed to many spores; however infection is uncommon.
• There is never pus unless there is secondary infection, which is rare.
• Lesions usually cause very little pain. There is marked local oedema and localized adenopathy.
• Pulmonary anthrax is very rare but has a very poor prognosis. Intestinal anthrax may also occur when infected animals are eaten, generally in Third-World countries.
• Penicillin is effective treatment. The eschar may take several weeks to separate. The mortality is now about 0.8%.
• Person-to-person transmission does not occur.

MANDELL, BENNETT & DOLIN (1995) p. 1593

121. Pyogenic meningitis

ANSWERS: a b c e

NOTES

• In adults *Streptococcus pneumoniae* is the most frequent organism causing pyogenic meningitis. Meningococcal meningitis is predominantly a disease of children and young adults (<10% of meningococcal meningitis occurs in those aged >45 years). *Haemophilus influenzae* is the commonest cause of meningitis between the neonatal period and 6 years of age.
• *H. influenzae* infection tends to run a subacute course, especially in children. Subdural effusions may develop, features of which include persistence of pyrexia beyond 72 h after initiation of therapy.
• Meningitis caused by Gram-negative bacteria (excluding *H. influenzae*) has increased significantly over the last 20 years. Head trauma and neurosurgery are the most common precipitating factors. *Klebsiella* is the most frequent organism implicated.
• In >80% of CSF samples which prove positive on culture the

organism can be identified on Gram stain. Latex agglutination can be used to identify pneumococcus, meningococcus and *Haemophilus*.

• Lumbar puncture reveals raised pressure, a polymorphonuclear leukocytosis, raised protein and low glucose levels.

MANDELL, BENNETT & DOLIN (1995) p. 741
WALTON (1993) p. 276

122. Diffuse fibrotic lung disease
ANSWERS: b c d

NOTES

• Causes of fibrotic lung disease include fibrosing alveolitis (Hamman–Rich), pulmonary scleroderma, polyarteritis nodosa, sarcoidosis, pulmonary berylliosis, asbestosis, extrinsic allergic alveolitis (e.g. farmer's lung) and lymphatic carcinomatosis.

• Predominant features include dyspnoea and hyperventilation. Lung function testing reveals a restrictive defect with reduced vital capacity, total lung capacity and compliance. There is hypoxia (only in association with exercise in the early stages), but the arterial Pco_2 level is normal or reduced. Diffuse radiographic abnormality is unusual.

• Reduction of single-breath carbon monoxide transfer is an early feature in fibrotic lung disease, predominantly due to a disturbance of ventilation and perfusion ratios. The forced expiratory volume in 1 s/forced vital capacity ratio is characteristically normal.

• Gallium scanning is abnormal in pulmonary fibrosis but is non-specific.

• In Hamman–Rich-type fibrosing alveloitis, bronchoalveolar lavage reveals an increased cell number, predominantly neutrophils and eosinophils. There is no consistent association with any specific HLA-A or B locus.

CROFTON & DOUGLAS (1989) pp. 130, 1004

123. Water balance
ANSWER: all incorrect

NOTES

• Approximately 100 ml of glomerular filtrate is produced every minute and 60–70% of this is reabsorbed in the proximal tubule.

• The descending limb of the loop of Henle is highly permeable to water, while the ascending limb is highly impermeable.

• Fluid in the descending tubule becomes increasingly hypertonic as water passes to the hyperosmolar extracellular fluid. The tonicity then falls progressively as the fluid passes up the ascending limb of the loop of Henle. Fluid entering the distal convoluted tubule is hypotonic.

• In the absence of AVP the distal convuluted tubule and collecting ducts are impermeable to water, but in the presence of AVP water is permitted to pass across the established concentration gradients and the intraluminal fluid thus becomes concentrated.

DEGROOT (1995) p. 1685

124. Constrictive pericarditis
ANSWERS: a b c d e

NOTES
• Cardiac failure, unaccompanied by severe dyspnoea, and often associated with ascites and congestive hepatomagaly, is characteristic of constrictive pericarditis. There is typically relatively little ankle oedema.

• Though the liver is commonly enlarged, it is not pulsatile.

• The jugular venous pressure is elevated and rises further on inspiration, in contrast to the normal fall seen on inspiration (Kussmaul's sign). Kussmaul's sign is not seen with acute tamponade. There is a marked 'y' descent of the jugular venous pressure when the tricuspid valve opens due to abnormally rapid early diastolic filling (Friedreich's sign; not seen with acute tamponade). The venous pressure rapidly returns to the previous elevated level and there is little further rise due to atrial contraction ('a' wave).

• The restricted pericardium causes an abrupt end to ventricular filling during diastole and a loud third heart sound (and knock).

• Pulsus paradoxus is characteristic in constrictive pericarditis (but is more marked in cases of acute tamponade). Kussmaul's sign may occur in severe heart failure and pulsus paradoxus in severe asthma.

• Atrial fibrillation develops in about 20% of cases. A decreased QRS voltage and T-wave changes on electrocardiography are very common.

• There is elevation and equalization of diastolic pressures in all four cardiac chambers.

BRAUNWALD (1992) p. 1482

125. Aortic dissection
ANSWERS: b c d

NOTES
• Dissecting aneurysm of the aorta results when a tear develops in the weakened media, usually a few centimetres above the aortic valve. There is extravasation of blood between the layers of the aortic wall. Proximal extension results in distortion of the aortic valve or valve ring and aortic regurgitation. Rupture into the pericardium is the commonest cause of death in cases of dissecting aneurysm.
• Cystic medial degeneration is a common factor in cases of aortic dissection. Predisposing conditions include:
(a) hypertension (present in over 50% of cases)
(b) coarctation of the aorta
(c) Marfan's syndrome (dissecting aortic aneurysm is the commonest cause of early death in these patients)
(d) Ehlers–Danlos syndrome
(e) pregnancy.
• Separation of the calcified aortic knuckle by >1 cm from the adventitial border of the aorta on chest X-ray is virtually pathognomonic of dissection.
• Syphilitic aortitis does not appear to predispose to aortic dissection. Although homocystinuria has certain features similar to those of Marfan's syndrome, dissecting aortic aneurysm is not associated.
• Transoesophageal ultrasound is currently the diagnostic modality of choice in suspected aortic dissection, although angiography remains the gold standard.
• Emergency medical treatment includes reduction of blood pressure and reduction of the ejection velocity of blood (thus reducing shearing forces). β-Blockade effectively reduces blood velocity. Surgery is optimal management for proximal dissections while opinion is less clear for distal dissections.

BRAUNWALD (1992) p. 1535
SCRIVER et al. (1989) pp. 2824, 2833

126. Splitting of the second heart sound
ANSWERS: a b c

NOTES
• Splitting of the second heart sound occurs as a result of the aortic valve closing slightly earlier than the pulmonary. This splitting is increased during inspiration, especially in children.
• Wide fixed (not varying with respiration) splitting of the second sound is a characteristic finding in atrial septal defect.
• Wide splitting of the second sound (which varies with respiration) occurs if the aortic valve closes early, as in the presence of ventricular septal defect or mitral regurgitation, or if the pulmonary valve closure is delayed, as in pulmonary valve stenosis or right bundle branch block.
• Wide splitting of the second sound does not occur in association with pulmonary hypertension unless there is associated right heart failure or right bundle branch block. In pulmonary hypertension the width of splitting is typically reduced.
• Reversed splitting of the second sound occurs when the pulmonary valve closes before the aortic valve.
• Reversed splitting is increased in width during expiration. It occurs in association with delayed aortic valve closure in aortic stenosis, left bundle branch block, HOCM, severe hypertension, patent ductus arteriosus and left heart failure. An alternative cause is early closure of the pulmonary valve as occurs in type B Wolff–Parkinson–White syndrome.

BRAUNWALD (1992) p. 30

127. Predisposition to large-bowel carcinoma
ANSWERS: a b d e

NOTES
• Large-bowel adenomatous polyps are not present at birth in FPC but multitudes develop throughout the colon, with occasionally a few in the terminal ileum. They are premalignant and carcinoma of the colon is a usual development before 40 years of age. Occasionally there is no family history of the condition.
• Multiple adenomatosis of the colon is a feature of Gardner's syndrome: the colonic adenomas are premalignant. Other features of

this syndrome include osteomas and soft-tissue tumours (sebaceous cysts, lipomas, etc.). Both FPC and Gardner's syndrome are dominantly inherited.

• The increased incidence of large-bowel carcinoma in ulcerative colitis is well-recognized, especially in association with diffuse long-standing disease. The increased incidence of colonic carcinoma begins after 7 years of disease and rises by 10% per decade to a maximum of 30%.

• Peutz–Jeghers syndrome is associated with multiple hamartomatous polyps of the small bowel (though a few may occur in the stomach and large bowel) and mucocutaneous pigmentation. Malignant change is rare but there is considered to be a slightly increased risk.

• The majority of carcinomas of the large bowel appear to develop from pre-existing adenomas which dedifferentiate as they enlarge.

• Ménétrier's disease is associated with giant hypertrophy of the gastric rugae, usually gastric hyposecretion and protein-losing enteropathy. Gastrin levels are usually normal. Up to 10% of cases may develop carcinoma of the stomach. Carcinoma of the large bowel is not associated.

SLEISENGER & FORDTRAN (1993) p. 1460

128. Leptospirosis
ANSWERS: b c d e

NOTES
• Fever headache, myalgia, conjunctivitis and meningism are prominent features of leptospirosis. In more severe cases hepatorenal failure with jaundice, impaired consciousness and bleeding diathesis may develop (Weil's disease).

• The CSF in patients with meningism usually shows a lymphocytosis, particularly in the later stages.

• Thrombocytopenia is common (>50%) and disseminated intravascular coagulation may occur.

• In contrast to the leucopenia usually seen in viral hepatitis, there is usually a polymorphonuclear leucocytosis in leptospirosis.

• *Leptospira* may be cultured from the blood during the first week of infection. During the second week blood culture is negative but serological tests become positive.

• *Leptospira* are sensitive to penicillin, and early administration of this antibiotic may influence the course of severe disease.

MANDELL, BENNETT & DOLIN (1995) p. 1813

129. Hyperuricaemia
ANSWERS: a b c e

NOTES
• Hyperuricaemia may result from increased formation or decreased excretion of uric acid.
• Increased formation occurs in:
(a) enzyme disorders (causing marked hyperuricaemia at an early age)
(b) Lesch–Nyhan syndrome
(c) hypoxathine-guanine phsphoribosyl-transferase deficiency
(d) type I glycogen storage disease (von Gierke's)
(e) superactive variants of phosphoribosylpyrophosphatate synthetase
(f) increased nucleoprotein turnover (e.g. myeloproliferative disease, polycythaemia, psoriasis)
(g) high dietary purine intake
(h) Down's syndrome.
• Decreased urate excretion occurs in:
(a) renal failure
(b) diuretic use
(c) therapy with uricostatic drugs
(d) lactic acidosis (including that associated with acute alcohol intoxication)
(e) ketosis (including that associated with starvation)
(f) lead poisoning.
• Xanthinuria is a rare condition associated with a low serum urate concentration and urinary excretion of xanthine and hypoxanthine.

SCRIVER *et al.* (1989) pp. 300, 965, 1085

130. Reiter's syndrome
ANSWERS: a c d

NOTES
• Reiter's disease is characterized by the classical triad of arthritis,

urethritis and conjunctivitis. It may follow an attack of chlamydial urethritis (non-specific urethritis, or NSU), or occasionally an attack of dysentery.

• In the UK, Reiter's syndrome usually follows sexually acquired urethritis; it is very much more commonly seen in males (predominantly 16–35 years).

• Reiter's syndrome may follow bacillary dysentery. Urethritis is frequently seen in the postdysenteric form, and diarrhoea often occurs when the disease follows an attack of NSU.

• There is an acute arthritis which is usually transient, predominantly involving the knees and ankles. Commonly four to five joints are affected asymmetrically. There is a marked polymorphonuclear leucocytosis in the synovial fluid. Calcaneal spurs are associated; they are typically large and fluffy on X-ray.

• Circinate balanitis is characteristic. It is equally frequent when the disease follows NSU or dysentery.

• Keratoderma blennorrhagica more frequently occurs when the disease follows NSU than dysentery. It most frequently involves the soles and may involve the nails.

• 75% of patients with Reiter's syndrome are found to be HLA B27-positive.

• Recurrence of Reiter's syndrome is common and occurs in about 60% of cases; this is often associated with infection, usually non-venereal. Chronic peripheral arthritis (predominantly metatarsophalangeal), sacroiliitis or ankylosing spondylitis may develop. Episcleritis, uveitis and cardiac defects (conduction defects and aortic valve incompetence) may occur in chronic disease.

• Chronic antimicrobial therapy may be effective in *Chlamydia*-induced reactive arthritis but not for postdysenteric cases.

KELLEY *et al.* (1993) p. 961

131. Chronic lymphatic leukaemia
ANSWERS: a b c d

NOTES
• CLL is characterized by progressive clonal expansion of long-lived, immunologically incompetent lymphocytes, 95% of which have B-cell morphology. A small minority of patients (about 5%) who have T-cell

morphology, pronounced neutropenia and skin involvement have a poor survival (<2 years).

• Males are more frequently affected (60–75% of cases). It is the commonest form of leukaemia seen in old age: it rarely occurs before 20 years of age.

• The leucocyte count is typically much raised (mean 93×10^9/l). There is a generalized lymphadenopathy which is usually symmetrical, 'rubbery' and painless.

• Skin lesions include local infiltration, generalized infiltration (*l'homme rouge*, usually associated with intense itching) and vesicobullous lesions. All are rare. Splenomegaly is an early feature in over 90% of patients.

• Significant hypogammaglobulinaemia occurs in 50% of cases, with predominant reduction of IgM. Some 5% show a clear monoclonal band on electrophoresis. Delayed hypersensitivity reactions to commonly used testing substances are reduced. Up to 20% of cases are complicated by herpes zoster, which may become generalized. There is a marked liability to infection and chest infections are very common.

• Vaccination with vaccinia is contraindicated in CLL since vaccinia gangrenosum and generalized vaccinia are significant risks.

• 30% of cases of CLL have a positive Coombs test but only 30% of these have a significant autoimmune haemolytic anaemia.

• Acute lymphoblastic transformation occurs very rarely (<2%) in CLL. Development of a diffuse histiocytic lymphoma (Richter's syndrome) occurs in about 10% of cases.

• Steroids result in rapid resolution of symptoms but further increase the risk of infection.

LEE *et al.* (1993) p. 751

DEVITA, HELLMAN & ROSENBERG (1993) p. 1965

132. Drug-induced lupus erythematosus
ANSWER: d

NOTES

• Drug-induced lupus erythematosus syndrome is most frequently associated with hydralazine, procainamide, isoniazid, chlorpromazine and methlydopa treatment. Many other drugs have been occasionally incriminated.

• In contrast to the idiopathic type of lupus erythematosus, the drug-induced variety does not show a great female preponderance.
• Renal and cerebral involvement are rarely features of the drug-induced syndrome.
• Most cases develop some months after the drug is initiated. The majority of cases resolve when the drug is withdrawn
• Most patients taking procainamide develop antinuclear antibodies but few develop a lupus syndrome.
• Antibodies to double-stranded DNA and Sm are almost invariably absent in cases of drug-induced lupus syndrome (in contrast to the presence of these antibodies in idiopathic SLE). Antibodies to histones are common in drug-induced lupus (90%) but are uncommon in spontaneous lupus (25%).
• The serum complement level is usually normal in drug-induced lupus erythematosus syndrome.

KELLEY *et al.* (1993) p. 1035

133. Lyme disease
ANSWER: C

NOTES
• Lyme disease is a multisystem disease which involves skin, central CNS, heart and joints.
• The spirochaete *Borrelia burgdorferi* is the aetiological agent and *Ixodes* ticks are the vector.
• The disease usually begins with a localized skin infection with a characteristic expanding skin lesion (erythema migrans) from which *B. burgdorferi* can be cultured. Without treatment spontaneous resolution of skin lesions usually occurs within 4 weeks. (Erythema marginatum is characteristic of rheumatic fever.)
• Disseminated infection subsequently develops with annular skin lesions, attacks of headache and neck stiffness, migratory polyarthritis and fatigue. Meningitis with cranial (especially facial) and peripheral neuropathy is associated.
• CSF shows an elevated protein and lymphocyte count.
• Cardiac involvement occurs in 5% and atrioventricular block is the commonest manifestation (when third-degree it is usually of short duration and does not require permanent pacing).
• In chronic cases longer bouts of oligoarticular joint inflammation

occur. In rare cases encephalomyelitis may occur (often in association with peripheral neuropathy).

• Serological testing (enzyme-linked immunosorbent assay) is the normal method of diagnosis.

• *B. burgdorferi* is only moderately sensitive to penicillin but is sensitive to tetracyclines, ampicillin and third-generation cephalosporins. Treatment should be prolonged (30 days).

KELLEY *et al.* (1993) p. 1484

134. Ankylosing spondylitis
ANSWER: C

NOTES

• >90% of cases of ankylosing spondylitis have the HLA B27 tissue type. Prevalence of HLA-B27 is low in Japanese people (<1%) .The risk for HLA-B27-positive individuals of developing ankylosing spondylitis is 1–2%.

• Ankylosing spondylitis is at least four times more common in males.

• Ankylosing spondylitis is characterized by backache and stiffness which are more prominent in the early morning and improved by exercise. Some 10% present with first symptoms before puberty.

• About 20% of cases present with a peripheral arthritis (especially involving the lower limb). Peripheral joint involvement occurs at some time in >30% of cases of ankylosing spondylitis.

• Anterior uveitis occurs in 20–40% of cases; it is usually unilateral. It may precede symptoms of ankylosing spondylitis.

• Aortic valve regurgitation is a rare complication of severe disease. Cardiomegaly and conduction defects may occur.

• Apical lung fibrosis, sometimes with cavitation, is a rare association of ankylosing spondylitis. Amyloid may occur in long-standing disease.

• In advanced cases spinal fractures, particularly of the cervical spine, may occur following minimal trauma and result in severe spinal cord damage.

KELLEY *et al.* (1993) p. 943

135. Spider telangiectasia
ANSWER: d

NOTES
• Vascular 'spiders' are associated with cirrhosis (especially alcoholic); they may also occur in normal individuals (particularly children), transiently in viral hepatitis, during pregnancy and rarely in rheumatoid arthritis.
• There is a central dilated arteriole, which may be elevated above the skin and become pulsatile. Pressure results in blanching.
• Lesions may resolve if liver function improves; however, development of new lesions is very suggestive of deterioration of function.
• 'Spider' telangiectasias occur in the area drained by the superior vena cava. They rarely occur below the level of the nipples.

SHERLOCK & DOOLEY (1993) p. 79

136. *Cryptococcus neoformans*
ANSWERS: b c

NOTES
• *Cryptococcus neoformans* is an encapsulated yeast-like fungus which grows in pigeon faeces but does not cause infection in the birds.
• Infection appears to occur after aerosol inhalation of the organism.
• Cryptococci activate the alternative complement pathway but complement is not present in CSF, which may predispose to the CNS localization of cryptococcal lesions.
• Acute presentations are more common in those with HIV infection.
• Cryptococcal infection usually presents with CNS symptoms and signs. Most patients have minimal or no neck rigidity. Cranial nerve lesions occur in about 20% of cases. Seizures are a late feature.
• Cryptococcal pneumonitis is usually mild or asymptomatic in normal individuals but may be severe and progresssive in HIV-infected patients.
• In cases with CNS involvement the CSF is almost invariably abnormal with increased pressure, decreased glucose, increased protein and an increased, predominantly lymphocytic, white-cell count. The organism may be seen on India ink smears or cultured.

MANDELL, BENNETT & DOLIN (1995) p. 2331

137. Zollinger–Ellison syndrome
ANSWERS: b d e

NOTES

• Inappropriately raised gastrin (a fasting level of >1000 pg/ml) is diagnostic of the Zollinger–Ellison syndrome (raised gastrin levels in association with high gastric acidity). High gastrin levels are also associated with atrophic gastritis, renal failure and occur after massive bowel resection.

• Both secretin and calcium infusion may be used to stimulate gastrin secretion in equivocal cases. Since basal acid secretion is enhanced in the Zollinger–Ellison syndrome, stimulation by pentagastrin classically increases acid output <40% above basal levels (however, this test is not diagnostic).

• Primary G-cell hyperplasia is a very rare cause of inappropriate gastrin hypersecretion.

• Diarrhoea and steatorrhoea may occur (due to mucosal damage, inactivation of lipase and precipitation of bile salts, by acid). Inhibition of intrinsic factor activity by the low intestinal pH may lead to B_{12} deficiency.

• Barium meal or gastroscopy may reveal gastric mucosal hypertrophy (also seen in Ménétrier's disease) or peptic ulceration. Distal duodenal or jejunal ulcertaion is virtually diagnostic of the Zollinger–Ellison syndrome.

• Most gastrinomas are located in the pancreas and two-thirds are malignant. Many are multifocal or metastatic at operation, making gastrectomy the usual treatment of choice. Some 25% of cases are associated with the MEN I syndrome and treatment of associated hyperparathyroidism may also relieve gastric symptoms.

• H_2-receptor blockade or omeprazole may be used therapeutically.

SLEISENGER & FORDTRAN (1993) p. 679
DEGROOT (1995) p. 2884

138. Migraine
ANSWERS: a b c d

NOTES

• Migraine is a paroxysmal disorder classically associated with visual or other cerebral disturbance, followed by unilateral headache and vomiting.

• Homonymous hemianopia is a characteristic migrainous visual disturbance. Resolution usually occurs within 20 min but may persist.

• Paraesthesiae, numbness and weakness may also occur (less commonly). Aphasia, usually expressive, is occasionally associated.

• The headache usually begins focally and spreads to involve the whole of one side of the head (occasionally the whole head). Stooping or straining aggravates the headache. Nausea and vomiting are usually associated.

• In ophthalmoplegic migraine there are recurrent attacks of headache associated with paralysis of one or more of the oculomotor nerves. The ophthalmoplegia persists and tends to become permanent after frequent attacks. Some such attacks may be caused by an intracerebral aneurysm.

• Horner's syndrome is a rare complication of frequent attacks.

• Attacks tend to become less severe and frequent with age, though there may be an exacerbation at the time of the menopause.

WALTON (1993) p. 130

139. Tamoxifen
ANSWER: C

NOTES
• Approximately 33% of cases of metastatic carcinoma of the breast will respond to tamoxifen therapy.

• Oestrogen receptor (ER)-positive patients show a 50–60% response rate. Tumours which are also progesterone-sensitive (PGR) show a higher response (65–75%).

• Only 5–10% of receptor-negative tumours respond.

• The level of ER is unrelated to the duration of response.

• Tamoxifen does not suppress ovulation in 50% of patients.

• Surgical oophorectomy is the treatment of choice in premenopausal patients with metastatic breast carcinoma while tamoxifen is the recommended first-line treatment in postmenopausal patients.

DEVITA, HELLMAN & ROSENBERG (1993) p. 1315

140. Mumps

ANSWERS: a d

NOTES

• In mumps, parotitis (pain and swelling), fever and malaise are usual. There is clear discharge from the parotid duct. Purulent discharge is indicative of suppurative parotitis.

• Subclinical infection is common, and is estimated to occur in about 30% of cases. Infection is rare in children aged less than 1 year.

• Before puberty mumps is rarely complicated by orchitis. Orchitis complicates about 20% of infections in adult males, usually developing as the parotid swelling is resolving. Orchitis is bilateral in 16–30% of cases. Sterility appears to be an infrequent outcome; testicular atrophy is more common.

• A lymphocytic meningitis, usually mild, occurs. The meningitis may develop in the absence of parotitis but usually occurs some days after the parotitis. Encephalitis is rare.

• The virus may be cultured from the saliva, urine and CSF, or the presence of virus demonstrated by the fluorescent antibody technique.

• Serological tests may be used to establish the diagnosis.

MANDELL, BENNETT & DOLIN (1995) p. 1260

141. Analgesic nephropathy

ANSWERS: a d

NOTES

• Analgesic nephropathy is characterized by chronic interstitial nephritis and renal papillary necrosis caused by excessive and prolonged consumption of analgesic mixtures.

• All cases have a disproportionate reduction of urinary concentrating ability and GFR is reduced in 80% of cases.

• There is a disproportionate systemic acidosis and renal tubular acidosis occurs in 10% of cases.

• Urinary tract infections occur in up to 60% and are a late complication.

• 35–40% of cases have haematuria.

• Significant proteinuria (>300 mg/day) occurs in 40–50% of cases

but nephrotic syndrome is unusual. Proteinuria is more common in those with poor renal function.
• Both hypertension and renal calculi are common.
• There is an increased risk of developing transitional cell carcinomas of the uroepithelium in analgesic abusers.

SCHRIER & GOTTSCHALK (1993). p. 1104

142. Paracetamol poisoning
ANSWERS: c e

NOTES
• Paracetamol is metabolized in the liver forming a toxic intermediate metabolite. This is conjugated with glutathione and thus detoxified. The ability to conjugate is overwhelmed in poisoning and toxic metabolite accumulates. This substance is an alkylating agent and causes centrilobular necrosis.
• Induction of liver enzymes by previous barbiturate and/or alcohol leads to greater intermediate metabolite production and potentiates toxicity.
• Ingestion of 25 g of paracetamol by an adult is likely to lead to hepatic necrosis. Children appear to be relatively less susceptible.
• Coma does not occur (before hepatic failure develops) unless other drugs have been taken.
• Paracetamol is not incriminated as a cause of haemolysis (in contrast to phenacetin).
• Vomiting and hepatic tenderness precede liver failure, which develops after 4–6 days. Features then include hypoglycaemia, prolonged PT, hyperventilation, jaundice, coma and acute renal failure.
• Acute renal failure may occur in association with hepatic failure or in isolation. Paracetamol in toxic quantities has antidiuretic activity.
• Acetylcysteine or methionine given within 12 h reduces the risk of liver damange.
• Hyperventilation is a feature of aspirin poisoning. It does not occur after paracetamol poisoning, except in association with hepatic failure.

GILMAN et al. (1990) p. 658

143. Varicella

ANSWER: c

NOTES
• The rash of varicella changes from macular to papular then to vesicles (generally superficial). The lesions then become pustular and crusting occurs. The rash is centripetal; however peripheral lesions occur and may develop on the palms and soles (as in smallpox).
• There is rapid evolution of the lesions to the vesicular stage and cropping occurs (lesions at differing stages of development).
• There are almost always lesions present in the mouth in association with skin lesions.
• Vesicular fluid is highly infectious; however respiratory transmission is important and the disease is most infectious when lesions are present in the upper respiratory tract. Crusts do not appear to be infectious.
• Varicella pneumonia may be severe and associated with respiratory distress, chest pain, haemoptysis and often cyanosis. There may be diffuse nodular infiltration on the chest X-ray, which may leave residual miliary calcification.
• The disease tends to be more severe in adults and the newborn: congenital infection can occur. There is usually no significant prodromal period. When prodromal symptoms occur infection is likely to be severe.
• Patients maintained on long-term steroid therapy and those who are immunosuppressed (e.g. leukaemics) are prone to develop severe infection.

MANDELL, BENNETT & DOLIN (1995) p. 1153
CROFTON & DOUGLAS (1989) p. 179

144. Hepatitis A

ANSWERS: b d e

NOTES
• Spread of hepatitis A is usually by the faecal–oral route. Parenteral infection also occurs.
• The incubation period is usually between 15 and 40 days; that of hepatitis B is longer (30–80 days).
• Features of infection include anorexia, nausea, vomiting, malaise,

162

fever and upper abdominal discomfort. Anicteric infection appears common, especially in young children.

• In those cases which become icteric the picture is that of an intrahepatic cholestasis with elevated conjugated bilirubin levels in the serum. The stools become pale and the urine dark. Serum alkaline phosphatase levels are moderately elevated.

• Recovery is usual after about 10 days of illness. Complications include persistent cholestasis, relapsing hepatitis, subacute hepatitis and rarely fulminant hepatitis with hepatic failure.

• Cases are infectious for 2–3 days before and about a week after the development of jaundice.

• Gammaglobulin injection appears to afford reasonable protection against hepatitis A.

MANDELL, BENNETT & DOLIN (1995) p. 1006

145. Hypercalcaemia
ANSWERS: a c d e

NOTES
• Primary and tertiary hyperparathyroidism are associated with hypercalcaemia. Secondary hyperparathyroidism is a physiological response to hypocalcaemia: it is not associated with hypercalcaemia.

• Hyperparathyroidism is the commonest cause of hypercalcaemia; malignancy is the second (together accounting for 90% of cases). Other causes include excessive vitamin D action and excessive bone turnover.

• Neoplasia may cause hypercalcaemia either due to bone metastases or, less commonly, as a result of tumour production of a substance with parathyroid hormone-like activity. This is usually associated with either a squamous carcinoma of the bronchus or a hypernephroma.

• Sarcoidosis is associated with vitamin D sensitivity and may lead to hypercalcaemia (usually in chronic sarcoidosis).

• Vitamin D intoxication leads to hypercalcaemia (due to bone reabsorption, reduced renal calcium clearance and increased intestinal calcium absorption).

• Milk-alkali syndrome results from excessive consumption of absorbable antacids with mild or calcium-rich foods. It is characterized by hypercalcaemia with renal failure, and normal phosphate levels.

163

• Thyrotoxicosis may cause mild hypercalcaemia (rarely severe). Transient hypercalcaemia is a feature of acute adrenal failure.

• Prolonged immobilization of patients may lead to hypercalcaemia, especially in those with high rates of bone turnover (e.g. Paget's disease).

• Idiopathic hypercalcaemia of infancy is a rare condition often associated with multiple congenital cardiovascular malformations.

• Lithium therapy appears to increase PTH secretion and has been associated with hypercalcaemia which resolves when the drug is stopped.

• If venous stasis is prolonged before the blood sample is obtained the plasma protein and calcium values may be falsely elevated.

DEGROOT (1995) p. 1081

146. Rabies
ANSWER: a

NOTES

• The incubation period of rabies is usually between 1 and 3 months. It is generally shorter after bites to the head and neck.

• The virus is of the RNA type with an affinity for the neurons of the CNS and mucus-secreting glands.

• There is malaise, fever and headache with pain and paraesthesiae spreading up the affected limb. Pupillary dilation and salivation precede the stage of excitement with apprehension and paralysis of the palate and limbs (at this stage hydrophobia may be evident). Progression to coma, convulsions and death then occurs.

• There is degeneration of neurons with characteristic inclusion bodies termed Negri bodies (absent in up to 30% of cases).

• Cats, and other carnivores, may be infected and transmit the infection to humans, though less frequently than is the case with dogs. Vampire bats transmit infection to cattle in South America.

• Human diploid cell vaccine appears the safest vaccine and is highly effective if administered before or shortly after exposure to the virus. Hyperimmune antirabies serum (from horse) has also been shown to be effective. Neither vaccine nor immunoglobulin appears to influence the course once clinical features develop, and death ensues (with very rare exceptions).

MANDELL, BENNETT & DOLIN (1995) p. 1291

147. Iron deficiency
ANSWERS: a b c

NOTES
• Absorption of inorganic iron is profoundly impaired in patients with achlorhydria
• Mean corpuscular volume (MCV) and MCH values are reduced. The mean corpuscular haemoglobin concentration (MCHC) is only rarely abnormal when the MCV and MCH are normal. It tends to be the last to fall as the deficiency worsens.
• Reticulocytes are normal or slightly increased, rarely decreased.
• Anisocytosis is an important early sign. Both anisocytosis and poikilocytosis are characteristic.
• The platelet count is characteristically raised, often to about twice the normal level.
• Total iron-binding capacity (TIBC) is usually increased and saturation of transferrin is always reduced. Serum ferritin levels are reduced.
• Basophilic stippling is a pronounced feature of thalassaemia and of sideroblastic anaemia but not of iron-deficiency anaemia.

LEE *et al.* (1993) pp. 797, 808

148. Cystic fibrosis
ANSWERS: b c d e

NOTES
• Cystic fibrosis is an autosomal recessive condition affecting exocrine glands which produce excessively viscous mucus and sweat with a high sodium concentration. The condition is much more common among whites than among the other racial groups.
• In cystic fibrosis the concentration of both sodium and chloride in the sweat is in excess of 70 mmol/l and sweat testing is both sensitive and specific. However, levels are much less reliable in adults since high levels may occur in healthy individuals. In contrast to the normal situation, sweat electrolyte concentrations do not fall after administration of aldosterone or fluorocortisone in patients with cystic fibrosis; this aids diagnosis.
• Heterozygotes are asymptomatic and have normal sweat electrolytes. Gene probes may be used for prenatal diagnosis using chorionic biopsy material.

• The viscid mucus in the respiratory tract causes bronchial obstruction and atelectasis with secondary infection. Bronchiectasis, fibrosis and emphysema develop. Clubbing is common and 15% have associated hypertrophic osteoarthropathy.

• Chronic sinus infection is a common association. Nasal polyps, which are normally rare during childhood, often occur in association with cystic fibrosis (30%). Haemoptysis complicates 50%.

• 10% of cases of cystic fibrosis present in the neonatal period with meconium ileus (often associated with volvus); rectal prolapse is common in older children. Albumin, not normally present in the stool, is found in stools from children with cystic fibrosis. Diabetes occurs in 12% and cirrhosis in 3%.

• Malabsorption develops in 80% of cases due to pancreatic insufficiency. The pancreatic secretion is excessively viscous and the trypsin level is low.

• A portal fibrosis which may progress to a multilobular cirrhosis is associated but usually remains asymptomatic. An elevated α-fetoprotein level is common.

• Most males with cystic fibrosis are aspermic; the vas deferens is frequently absent or atrophic. Females are usually infertile.

CROFTON & DOUGLAS (1989) p. 784

149. Signs of lobar consolidation
ANSWERS: a b c

NOTES
• Where consolidation is present chest movement on that side may be reduced. The percussion note is dull, sometimes 'stony' dull. The vocal fremitus is normal or increased, in contrast to the reduced vocal fremitus associated with pleural effusion.

• There may be a pleural rub overlying an area of consolidation, especially in association with pleuritic pain.

• Bronchial breathing may be present: it is a harsh or blowing sound with a duration of the expiratory noise as long as or longer than the inspiratory (it is similar in nature to the sound heard by listening directly over the trachea).

• In addition to consolidation, bronchial breathing may occur in association with both pulmonary collapse and a thin layer of pleural fluid overlying the lung.

• Whispering pectoriloquy is present in the same areas as bronchial breathing. They are inseparable signs.
• The trachea is not shifted when consolidation occurs since there is no mediastinal shift.

CROFTON & DOUGLAS (1989) p. 116

150. Guillain–Barré syndrome (acute idiopathic polyneuritis)
ANSWERS: b c

NOTES
• Guillain–Barré syndrome (acute idiopathic polyneuritis) produces a relatively symmetrical tetraparesis. Tendon reflexes are usually lost early in the disease.
• Paraesthesia of the toes (less commonly of the fingers) is the first neurological symptom in 75% of cases.
• 50% of patients have pain, usually of the back and buttocks.
• Presence of autonomic neuropathy cannot be predicted from the severity of motor or sensory neuropathy. Sudden cardiac death is a recognized complication.
• Conduction studies may be normal in early disease despite severe paralysis. Conduction block with reduced amplitude of the compound muscle action potential is the commonest finding in the first 2 weeks. Distal slowing of motor conduction occurs later.
• A subgroup of patients have axonal degeneration. These patients have a worse prognosis with prolonged weakness.
• A much raised albumin concentration in the CSF occurs in 80% of cases (>2 g/l). The cell count is generally normal. A slightly increased number of mononucleated cells occurs in 10% of cases. The high albumin concentration may lead to spontaneous clotting of samples of CSF.
• Plasma exchange has been shown to reduce the time before patients start to improve, and to reduce the requirement for assisted ventilation. Intravenous immunoglobulin also appears to be effective.

WALTON (1993) p. 599

151. Acclimatization to altitude
ANSWERS: a b

NOTES

• At altitude the partial pressure of oxygen is reduced in the inspired air. Adaptation to the chronic hypoxia occurs. Continuous habitation for centuries has occurred at 4200–4500 m.

• Acute adaptation involves an increase of the minute volume and hypocapnia, mediated by the peripheral chemoreceptors (which are sensitive to hypoxia). Initially the hyperventilation is reversible when oxygen is administered but becomes irreversible after 5–10 days.

• Ventilatory response to raised carbon dioxide levels is increased (a result of reduced bicarbonate levels, and thus buffering, in the CSF).

• Polycythaemia occurs, taking some months to develop fully.

• The oxygen affinity of the haemoglobin is reduced (the oxygen dissociation curve is shifted to the right), facilitating oxygen release to the tissue. The altered affinity is due to increased red-cell 2,3 DPG levels, production of which is stimulated by hypoxia.

CROFTON & DOUGLAS (1989) p. 61

152. *Mycoplasma pneumoniae*
ANSWERS: a b e

NOTES

• *Mycoplasma pneumoniae* is a mycoplasma. These are the smallest known free-living organisms (i.e. they grow on cell-free media).

• There is a peak rate of infection in the autumn and early winter. The majority of cases occur between childhood and 30 years of age. Only 3–10% of cases appear to develop pneumonia. *M. pneumoniae* infection has been implicated in 18% of cases of pneumonia.

• The incubation period is about 3 weeks. The features include headache, myalgia, pharyngitis, tracheobronchitis, pyrexia and dry cough. Sputum is usually scanty, mucoid or blood-stained. There may be retrosternal pain but this is seldom pleuritic and rigors are unusual. Pleural effusion is documented in 7% of cases.

• The white cell count is not elevated unless there is secondary bacterial infection.

• Haemolytic anaemia and meningism may develop in severe cases. Myocarditis, arthritis, urticarial rash and the Stevens–Johnson syndrome are recognized complications.

• Agglutinins to human group O red cells which are active under cold conditions (cold agglutinins) are present in up to 50% of cases. They are more frequently associated with severe cases. In a smaller proportion (30%) of cases agglutinins to a non-haemolytic streptococcus (streptococcus MG) are present, though this organism bears no common antigen with the mycoplasma and has no causal relationship with the disease.

• Mycoplasmal infection may be confirmed by serological testing, including complement fixation.

• A vaccine against *M. pneumoniae* is now available. The organism is sensitive to both tetracycline and erythromycin.

• A similar picture to that caused by *M. pneumoniae* infection is seen in legionnaire's disease. This disease is caused by a small Gram-negative coccobacillus. It is sensitive to erythromycin, but less so to tetracycline.

CROFTON & DOUGLAS (1989) p. 306

153. Immunoglobulin
ANSWERS: c d

NOTES
• Chemical separation of the polypeptide chains of immunoglobulin produces light chains common to all immunoglobulin classes and class-specific heavy chains.

• There are two types of light chains, termed κ and λ. Each immunoglobulin molecule has a four-chain structure with two light and two heavy chains.

• There are constant and variable regions of both heavy and light chains. The variable regions form the antigen-binding sites.

• Antibodies may be cleaved by papain into two Fab (fragment antigen binding) and one Fc (fragment crystalline) fragments.

• IgG is the major subclass of immunoglobulin accounting for about 75% of total immunoglobulin.

• The Fc fragment of IgG is responsible for C1q binding and complement activation (two juxtaposed IgG molecules are required for effective activation), the ability to bind to macrophages, and maternofetal transport of IgG.

• IgA in secretions is dimeric and is associated, via the Fc fragment, with a polypeptide chain—the secretory component (SC). It is the main immunoglobulin in exocrine secretions.

• IgM is the first immunoglobulin to be produced following antigenic challenge. Bound to cell membranes IgM is a powerful activator of complement. It does not cross the placenta. Monomeric IgM is the major antibody receptor on the cell walls of B lymphocytes for antigen recognition.

• IgE does not activate complement or cross the placenta. IgE binds with high affinity to a receptor on mast cells and circulating basophils.

LACHMANN *et al.* (1993) p. 149

154. Cerebrospinal fluid
ANSWER: b

NOTES
• The CSF is formed mainly by the choroid plexuses of the cerebral ventricles. It appears to result from both ultrafiltration and active secretion. The normal volume of CSF is about 130 ml.

• The normal lumbar CSF protein level is below 350 mg/l, which is very much lower than the plasma level of about 70 g/l. The albumin : globulin ratio is 8 : 1.

• The concentration of sodium is similar in both the CSF and plasma.

• The chloride concentration is normally 15–20 mmol/l higher in the CSF than in the plasma. However, chloride measurement in the CSF is of no clinical value.

• Elevated CSF IgG (oligoclonal) is associated with multiple sclerosis as is identification of P2 protein (a constituent of myelin) in CSF by immunoassay.

• The CSF is maintained at a pH of close to 7.33. This is somewhat lower than the blood pH.

• The glucose level in the CSF is normally 60–70% of that of the plasma. It is reduced below this level in tuberculous and carcinomatous meningitis and is usually very low in pyogenic meningitis.

WALTON (1993) p. 56

155. Aldosterone

ANSWER: all incorrect

NOTES

• Aldosterone is a steroid hormone secreted by the zona glomerulosa of the adrenal cortex.

• Aldosterone acts on the distal convoluted tubule promoting sodium retention (reabsorption) and resulting in potassium (and ammonium) excretion. When aldosterone secretion is prolonged the kidney 'escapes' from the sodium-retaining activity, and the potassium loss continues.

• The majority of the filtered sodium is reabsorbed in the proximal tubule. Only a small proportion passes to the distal tubule where reabsorption is under the influence of aldosterone.

• Reduced sodium intake enhances proximal reabsorption of sodium. Less sodium is delivered to the distal tubule to be reabsorbed under the influence of aldosterone. There is thus less potassium loss in the urine.

• Sodium retention leads to secondary retention of water. However, aldosterone has no direct action on water excretion.

• Aldosterone decreases the sodium and increases the potassium concentration of both sweat and saliva.

• Renin is secreted by the juxtaglomerular apparatus in the kidney (β-adrenergic blockade inhibits renin release). This is a major regulator of aldosterone secretion, through the mediation of angiotensin I and II. Potassium also appears to influence aldosterone secretion, low levels being inhibitory.

• ACTH injections do initially stimulate aldosterone secretion. However, the secretion rate falls to normal if administration is prolonged.

• After acute hypophysectomy in humans the aldosterone response to sodium depletion is unimpaired. However, after some years, there is little or no increase in aldosterone levels in response to sodium depletion.

DEGROOT *et al.* (1995) p. 1668

156. Antineutrophil cytoplasmic antibodies
ANSWERS: a d e

NOTES

• ANCAs occur in highest titre in cases of Wegener's granulomatosis and vasculitis in which necrotizing and crescentic glomerulonephritis is prominent.

• ANCAs are unusual in classical polyarteritis nodosa (PAN) and are rare in secondary vasculitis.

• A pattern of diffuse cytoplasmic staining (C-ANCA) is commonly seen in Wegener's granulomatosis.

• A perinuclear pattern of staining (P-ANCA) is associated with microscopic polyarteritis and cresentic glomerulonephritis. In the case of P-ANCA the antigen appears to be myeloperoxidase.

• Levels of ANCA correlate with disease activity and rises tend to occur before clinical features are evident, suggesting a cause-and-effect relationship.

SCHRIER & GOTTSCHALK (1993). p. 2097

157. α-Adrenergic stimulation
ANSWERS: a b

NOTES

• α-Adrenergic stimulation results in vasoconstriction, uterine contraction and pupillary dilation. There is inhibition of insulin secretion in response to a glucose load and stimulation of apocrine sweating in axillary areas. Phenylephrine is a selective α-receptor agonist, phenoxybenzamine a selective α-antagonist.

• β-Adrenergic stimulation results in cardiac stimulation and lypolysis. Practolol is a selective β-antagonist.

• β-Adrenergic stimulation results in bronchodilation and vasodilation. Salbutamol is a selective β-agonist.

• Intestinal smooth-muscle relaxation occurs in response to both α- and β-adrenergic stimulation. The receptor responsible for stimulation of glycogenolysis and gluconeogenesis is not yet clearly determined.

• Adenyl cyclase appears to accumulate intracellularly in response to β-sympathetic stimulation, and to be a mediator of activity.

DEGROOT et al. (1995) p. 1855

158. Metabolic effects of prolonged vomiting
ANSWERS: b c d e

NOTES
• In pyloric stenosis there is continued vomiting of acid gastric fluid, without loss of vomiting of alkaline duodenal fluid.
• There is hypovolaemia and a metatolic alkalosis (a result of H^+ and Cl^- loss; hypokalaemia is an additional factor contributing to alkalosis).
• The kidney is generally effective at removing excess bicarbonate from the body. However, renal bicarbonate excretion is inhibited by hypochloraemia, hypokalaemia and reduced glomerular filtration rate–all of which result from prolonged vomiting.
• Fluid and electrolyte replacement enables the kidney to excrete bicarbonate.
• In response to a metabolic alkalosis there is compensatory hypoventilation. This results in an increased carbonic acid concentration; however, this is produced in inadequate quantity to compensate for the alkalosis.
• During metabolic alkalosis where there is an associated hypokalaemia the kidney excretes an acid urine. This is inappropriate in the presence of a systemic alkalosis and is termed paradoxical aciduria.

SLEISENGER & FORDTRAN (1993) p. 518

159. Atrial myxoma
ANSWERS: a c

NOTES
• Myxomas are the commonest primary cardiac tumours (30–50%). The mean age for sporadic myxoma is 56 years and 70% are female.
• 86% occur in the left atrium (usually attached in the region of the fossa ovalis) and 90% are solitary.
• Clinical features include non-specific effects (e.g. pyrexia of unknown origin), embolization and interference with cardiac function.
• 7% of cases are familial. In these patients myxomas are often multiple and present earlier (mean age <30 years). Syndromes including myxomas have been described including NAME (naevi, atrial myxoma, myxoid neurofibroma, ephelides) and LAMB (lentigines, atrial myxoma and blue naevi).

173

• Following surgical resection recurrence rates are low (1–5%) in spontaneous cases.

BRAUNWALD (1992) p. 1451

160. Peripheral neuropathy
ANSWERS: a c d e

NOTES
• In demyelinating neuropathies conduction velocity is markedly delayed. If demyelination affects predominantly the proximal portion of the nerve then distal velocity may be preserved but the F-wave response will be prolonged (conduction to the cord and back).
• In axonal neuropathies conduction velocity may be normal but the evoked sensory or motor action potential is greatly reduced in amplitude.
• The sensory action potentials tend to be preserved in root lesions (where dorsal root ganglia are preserved) and this observation helps to distinguish them from plexus or peripheral nerve lesions.
• About 2 weeks after total transection of the nerve, fibrillation potentials develop in the innervated muscle. Fibrillation potentials do not occur in neuropraxia.
• Fasciculation potentials occurring spontaneously, indistinguishable from motor unit action potentials, occur in a setting of active denervation.

WALTON (1993) p. 558

161. Results of splenectomy
ANSWERS: a b c d e

NOTES
• Removal of the spleen from infants and young children renders them very susceptible to infection, especially overwhelming septicaemia (especially pneumococcal). The risk appears less when the operation is performed at an older age.
• After splenectomy a variable proportion of the red cells become target cells. They have an increased membrane lipid and surface area with abnromal resistance to saline haemolysis.
• The reticulocyte count is increased, there is an increased proportion

of misshapen circulation red cells and Howell–Jolly bodies (remnants of nuclear material), Heinz bodies (inclusions of denatured haemoglobin due to oxidative damage) and siderocytes appear. Nucleated red cells are seldom seen.

• An increased white-cell count is usual. Initially after operation this is of polymorphonuclear cells, but later the increase is of lymphocytes and monocytes.

• Platelets are increased, up to >1 million × 10^9/l after 7–12 days. Thereafter there is a fall towards more normal levels.

LEE *et al.* (1993) p. 316

162. Staphylococcal toxic shock syndrome
ANSWERS: b c d e

NOTES
• TSS is caused by toxin-producing staphylococci.
• >90% of normal healthy individuals have been demonstrated to have antibody to the TSS toxin TSST-1 while nearly all of the menstruation-associated cases have undetectable antibody to TSST-1 at the onset of TSS.
• Diagnostic criteria for TSS include:
(a) temperature >38.9°C
(b) systolic blood pressure <90 mmHg
(c) rash with subsequent desquamation (especially of the palms and soles)
(d) involvement of three or more of:
    vomiting or profuse diarrhoea
    severe myalgia or creatine phosphokinase greater than five times normal
    frank mucosal membrane hyperaemia
    renal insufficiency (creatinine greater than twice normal)
    hepatitis (bilirubin, serum glutamic oxaloacetic transaminase greater than twice normal)
    thrombocytopenia (<100 000/mm^3)
    disorientation without focal neurological signs.

MANDELL, BENNETT & DOLIN (1995) p. 1766

163. Subarachnoid rupture of a cerebral aneurysm
ANSWERS: a b c e

NOTES

• Sudden development of the symptoms and signs of meningeal irritation is the usual presentation of rupture. Unconsciousness occurs in about 50% of cases but may be brief.

• Retinal haemorrhage (subhyaloid or vitreous) may be associated (probably secondary to acute compression of the central vein of the retina). Papilloedema is uncommon and is usually slight.

• Red cells are present in the CSF for a week or more after subarachnoid haemorrhage. Xanthochromia develops within 12 h (due to the presence of yellow haemoglobin pigments). There is often a leucocytosis, usually predominantly of mononuclear cells.

• Without treatment 50% of patients die within the first month after rupture, half in the first day. Vascular malformations which bleed have a lower mortality and less chance of rebleeding than do aneurysms.

• Hydrocephalus complicates 10% of cases.

• After rupture, spasm of the artery on which the aneurysm is situated causing cerebral ischaemia occurs in 25% of cases and has a bad prognosis. Nimodipine may reduce the risk of spasm; volume expansion and induced hypertension may reverse neurological signs.

• The first day CT scan shows intracranial blood in over 90% of cases.

• Patients presenting with sudden headache who have a normal CT scan and CSF when examined within 2 weeks of the headache do not require additional angiography to rule out aneurysm. Those presenting more than 2 weeks after the event require four-vessel angiography to rule out the presence of aneurysm or vascular malformation.

• Saccular cerebral aneurysms tend to form at branching points on the circle of Willis: 40% on the anterior communicating artery, 25% on the middle cerebral artery, 30% on the posterior communicating artery and 5% on the posterior cerebral arterial circulation.

WALTON (1993) pp. 228, 248

164. Target cells

ANSWERS: b c d

NOTES

• On stained blood films, target cells have central and peripheral stained areas separated by a pallid ring. They tend to be flat in shape and to have lost the characteristic biconcave red-cell morphology.

• Target cells are abnormally resistant to saline haemolysis and this is a feature of haemoglobin C disease in which target cells are especially numerous.

• Target cells are common in thalassaemia (both homozygous and heterozygous), haemoglobin C and D disease and sickle-cell anaemia.

• Target cells are a constant and characteristic finding postsplenectomy and are also seen in liver disease.

• Target cells are prominent in LCAT deficiency.

• Spherocytes occur in autoimmune haemolytic anaemia and glucose-6-phosphatase deficiency. Target cells are not associated.

LEE *et al.* (1993) pp. 957, 982, 1010, 1173

165. Immunoglobulin A deficiency

ANSWERS: b c e

NOTES

• One in 600 caucasians is IgA-deficient, making this the most common immunodeficiency.

• 20% of patients with IgA deficiency have associated IgG subclass deficiency. This group have increased incidence of recurrent respiratory infections.

• 50–70% of patients with ataxia telangiectasia are IgA-deficient.

• Allergy and autoimmune disease may be increased in patients with IgA deficiency.

• There is a high incidence of antibodies to dietary ruminant proteins (milk proteins) in deficient subjects.

• Patients with IgA deficiency frequently develop antibodies to IgA and if they require antibody administration may require IgA-depleted immunoglobulin.

• There is no recognized association between IgA deficiency and duodenal ulceration.

LACHMANN *et al.* (1993) p. 1273

166. Visual pathway

ANSWERS: a c e

NOTES

• Division of optic nerve results in unilateral blindness. A midline lesion of the chiasma involves the decussating fibres and a bitemporal hemianopia results. When the chiasma is compressed from below (as by a pituitary tumour) the visual field defect is initially of the upper bitemporal quadrants.

• A homonymous hemianopia occurs, in association with a pituitary tumour, about half as often as a bitemporal hemianopia.

• The optic tract conveys fibres from the temporal side of the ipsilateral retina and the nasal side of the contralateral retina. A complete lesion of the optic tract therefore results in a contralateral (crossed) homonymous hemianopia. However lesions of the optic tracts are rarely complete.

• The optic tract runs to the lateral geniculate body where the fibres synapse. The efferent fibres emerge from the posterior limb of the internal capsule of the optic radiation and run to the occipital lobe.

• The fibres from the upper part of the retina run a direct course, but those from the lower retina run a longer course over the tip of the descending horn of the lateral ventricle. These lower fibres may be involved by a temporal lobe lesion, resulting in a visual field defect involving the upper part of the visual field (crossed homonymous superior quadrantic anopia).

• A parietal lesion is associated with a crossed inferior quadrantic anopia.

WALTON (1993) p. 79

167. Facial nerve

ANSWERS: c d e

NOTES

• The facial nerve is a purely motor nerve but is associated through part of its course by fibres which excite salivation and others which convey taste from the anterior two-thirds of the tongue.

• The nucleus of the facial nerve is situated in the ventral part of the tegmentum of the pons.

- The fibres pass backwards from the nucleus and loop around the sixth nerve nucleus. They then pass forwards again to emerge from the lateral aspect of the lower border of the pons on the medial side of the eighth nerve.
- The nerve passes through the cerebellopontine angle and into the internal acoustic meatus. It runs in the facial canal in the petrous temporal bone, and thence on the medial side of the middle ear. After turning down behind the middle ear the nerve emerges from the stylomastoid foramen.
- The geniculate ganglion is situated in the region of the middle ear. Here the nervus intermedius (which conveys secretory and gustatory fibres) joins the facial nerve. The ganglion contains the ganglion cells of the taste fibres (which are conveyed to the facial nerve by the chorda tympani).
- The greater petrosal nerve originates from the region of the geniculate ganglion. It gives fibres to the otic and pterygopalantine ganglia and is responsible for the stimulation of salivation.
- In the facial canal the nerve gives a branch to the stapedius muscle and receives the fibres of the chorda tympani.
- The facial nerve is the motor nerve to the facial muscles. It is the efferent part of the corneal reflex.

WALTON (1993) p. 106

168. Common peroneal nerve
ANSWERS: a b d

NOTES
- Division of the common peroneal nerve results in paralysis and wasting of the peronei and anterior tibial muscles. There is paralysis of dorsiflexion of the foot, resulting in footdrop.
- The power of eversion is lost and weak inversion is only possible with the foot in plantar flexion.
- A lesion above the lateral cutaneous branch causes anaesthesia of the lateral aspect of the dorsum of the foot and the anterolateral region of the lower leg (a lesion below the lateral cutaneous branch leads to anaesthesia only over the dorsum of the foot).
- The tibial nerve (medial popliteal) innervates the calf muscles and those of the sole of the foot. It also mediates the ankle and plantar reflexes.

• The common peroneal nerve is much more susceptible to injury than the tibial.

• The sensory distribution of the sciatic nerve is entirely below the level of the knee. The sciatic nerve innervates the hamstrings and the short head of the biceps femoris before dividing into the common peroneal and tibial nerves in the proximal part of the popliteal fossa.

• The common peroneal nerve is a particularly frequent site of a mononeuropathy (as, for example, may occur with diabetes of polyarteritis nodosa). In such cases sensory disturbance is usually minimal.

WALTON (1993) pp. 36, 588

169. Polycystic kidney disease
ANSWERS: a b c d e

NOTES

• ADPKD progresses to end-stage renal failure in about 50% of those affected. In about 60% of cases there is a positive family history (although ultrasound will reveal cysts in one or more family members in 90% of cases).

• ADPKD has a prevalence of 1:200 to 1:1000.

• A gene on the short arm of chromosome termed ADPKD-1 has been identified and accounts for approximately 90% of cases of ADPKD in the white population.

• Probes to genes linked to ADPKD-1 can be used in diagnosis but are not 100% accurate since genes can be separated during mitosis (crossover).

• In adults with polycystic kidney disease, abdominal or flank pain occurs in about 50%. Haematuria occurs in 30–50%. Fewer than 5% experience abdominal distension and bloating.

• Hypertension is associated in 70%. Urinary infections are more common and urinary calculi occur in up to 30%.

• Hepatic cysts occur in 30–60% of cases of ADPKD but hepatic failure or portal hypertension is extremely rare.

• Autosomal recessive polycystic kidney disease is usually discovered shortly after birth and results in end-stage renal disease in childhood.

SCHRIER & GOTTSCHALK (1993) p. 535

170. Wegener's granulomatosis
ANSWERS: a b c

NOTES
• Features of Wegener's granulomatosis include necrotizing granulomatous lesions of the respiratory tract, GN and vasculitis.
• The renal lesion is most commonly a rapidly progressive focal necrotizing GN but other lesions such as diffuse proliferative GN may also occur.
• Necrotizing and crescentic glomerulonephritis is typical.
• ANCAs, with the characteristic diffuse cytoplasmic staining (C-ANCA), are found in over 90% of cases and are related to disease activity.
• Slightly improved survival was associated with steroid use (from 20% 1-year survival to 34%) but cyclophosphamide increases 1-year survival to 90% and 5-year survival to 80%. Long-term addition of steroids appears to be of no advantage.
• Cyclophosphamide is optimally continued for 1 year after complete remission.

KELLEY *et al.* (1993) p. 1091
SCHRIER & GOTTSCHALK (1993) p. 2108

171. *Schistosoma haematobium*
ANSWERS: b e

NOTES
• The miracidia of *Schistosoma haematobium* infect living water snails from which the cercariae are liberated. The cercariae penetrate human skin and thence develop into adult worms.
• During the early stages of the disease there may be fever, malaise, myalgia and sometimes urticaria.
• The worms, of both sexes, develop in the vesical and pelvic venous plexuses. The worms may survive for many years.
• Eggs are released into the tissues and excite a granulomatous reaction. The characteristic terminal spined eggs are excreted in the urine. Haematuria is usual; it is classically terminal.
• The granulomatous reaction in the bladder wall progresses to fibrosis and calcification may eventually occur. Ureteric obstruction

may occur and the reduced bladder capacity results in increased frequency and precipitance of micturition.

• There is an increased incidence of carcinoma of the bladder.

• Eggs also circulate to the lungs where a granulomatous reaction occurs. This may result in cor pulmonale in severe cases but is more often associated with the other varieties of schistosomiasis (*S. mansoni* and *japonicum*).

• *S. haematobium* may be treated with metriphonate or niridazole.

• *S. haematobium* occurs in Africa and the Medditerranean region of the Middle East; it does not occur in the Far East.

MAEGRAITH (1989) p. 391

172. Secretin test
ANSWERS: b c e

NOTES

• Pancreatic exocrine function is tested by measuring the response to a standard stimulus. In the Lundh test, a test meal is given and the tryptic activity in the duodenal aspirate is measured. An alternative stimulus is intravenous secretin.

• Measurements may be made of the volume, enzyme concentration and the bicarbonate content of the aspirate. There is a wide range of normality for all of these values.

• In chronic pancreatitis volume, enzyme concentration and bicarbonate content are all classically reduced. The functional findings in cystic fibrosis are the same.

• The bicarbonate concentration of the aspirate is classically normal when a carcinoma partially obstructs the pancreatic duct. Unfortunately, values are usually normal when the tumour is in the body or tail of the pancreas.

• After vagotomy there is a slight diminution in the pancreatic response to a test meal. Vagal stimulation appears to result in a modest rise in the volume and enzyme content of the secretion.

• If cholecystokinin (CCK) is administered in addition to secretin then pancreatic secretion is enhanced; however, the diagnostic yield is not improved.

• Secretin results in a paradoxical increase in gastrin levels in patients with gastrinoma.

SLEISENGER & FORDTRAN (1993) pp. 686, 1593, 1660

173. Secretin

ANSWERS: a b c e

NOTES

• Secretin is a polypeptide hormone of 27 amino acids. It is released from the duodenal and upper jejunal mucosa in response to intraluminal acid (but not intraluminal glucose). Although vagal stimulation stimulates gastric acid production it has no direct action on secretin secretion.

• Secretin stimulates pancreatic water and bicarbonate secretion. It also enhances the secretion of pancreatic enzymes in response to vagal stimulation, inhibits gastrin and gastric acid release and enhances CCK-mediated gallbladder contraction.

• Secretin release is inhibited by somatostatin.

• At pharmacological levels secretin results in reduction of lower oesophageal sphincter tone and stimulation of insulin secretion.

DEGROOT (1995) p. 2873

174. Cholecystokinin

ANSWERS: d e

NOTES

• CCK is a polypeptide hormone. It is released from the duodenum and upper jejunum in response to intraluminal fat (especially unsaturated fatty acids of 10–18 carbon atom length) and amino acids such as phenylalanine and tryptophan.

• The vagus does not appear to be an important influence on CCK release, which is unimpaired after vagotomy.

• CCK stimulates gallbladder contraction and relaxation of the sphincter of Oddi. Other physiological functions of CCK include stimulation of pancreatic enzyme secretion, enhancement of secretion-stimulated pancreatic bicarbonate secretion, inhibition of gastric emptying and stimulation of small-bowel mobility.

• CCK is a major neurotransmitter and is distributed widely throughout the CNS.

• The gallbladder concentrates bile (up to 10 times) by active sodium transport. This mechanism does not appear to be regulated by hormonal or neural control.

DEGROOT (1995) p. 2872

175. Bronchopulmonary aspergillosis
ANSWERS: b c e

NOTES
• Bronchopulmonary aspergillosis usually occurs in those with asthma or complicates cystic fibrosis. Features include exacerbation of wheeze and cough associated with fever and malaise.
• It occurs predominantly in autumn and winter.
• Chest X-ray classically shows a patchy infiltrate often with associated segmental collapse.
• Eosinophilia is characteristic; specific precipitating IgG antibodies are present in 70% of patients and specific IgE antibodies are also associated.
• Affected patients exhibit an immediate reaction to skin testing to *Aspergillus fumigatus*
• (but *A. terreus*, which also causes disease, does not cross-react).
• Culture of *A. fumigatus* from the sputum is not diagnostic and occurs in normals (since spores are ubiquitous): demonstration of hyphae in sputum is diagnostic. Sputum is charactistically viscous and plugs or casts containing fungal hyphae are characteristic.
• Early treatment with steroids generally results in resolution, although some patients develop progressive disease with fibrosis and bronchiectasis. In these cases antifungal treatment is indicated.

CROFTON & DOUGLAS (1989) p. 461

176. Visceral leishmaniasis
ANSWERS: b e

NOTES
• Visceral leishmaniasis results from infection, predominantly of the reticuloendothelial cells, by *Leishmania donovani*. The vector is a sandfly of the *Phlebotomus* species.
• There is a reservoir of infection among small rodents.
• The incubation period varies from 2 weeks to longer than 18 months.
• There is an irregular fever; prostration and delirium are usual, as is progressive hepatosplenomegaly (the spleen may become huge). Lymphadenopathy is not generally associated.
• A leucopenia, with a relative mononucleosis, is characteristic.

Anaemia is usual; hypersplenism may develop. There is a low serum albumin and raised gammaglobulin. The albumin/globulin ratio is reversed (i.e. <1).

• The organism may be identified in the blood or samples of spleen, bone marrow and liver. The Leishmanin skin test is negative in active disease: it becomes positive as immunity develops.

• Treatment is by pentavalent antimonials or by pentamidine (a diamidine).

MAEGRAITH (1984) p. 189

177. Falciparum malaria
ANSWERS: b c d

NOTES

• Falciparum malaria has an incubation period of 8–15 days; prodromal symptoms are often severe. The *Anopheles* mosquito is the vector.

• The periods of well-being between bouts of fever, characteristic of the other varieties of malaria, are often absent in falciparum malaria. The fever often does not resolve between bouts. In a minority of cases a periodicity of fever develops, usually tertian or quotidian.

• A severe anaemia is common. There is usually a slight leucopenia.

• Vomiting and diarrhoea at the onset of disease are frequent. Herpes labialis is often associated. The spleen is enlarged and usually palpable after 10 days.

• Complications include cerebral malaria, hyperpyrexia, cardiovascular collapse (algid) and haemolysis (blackwater fever).

• Blackwater fever is associated with inadequate antimalarial therapy.

• Falciparum malaria may recur but rarely longer than 1 year after original infection.

• 4-Aminoquinolines (e.g. chloroquine) are schizonticidal (i.e. they eradicate the red-cell forms). Both proguanil and pyrimethamine (also 4-aminoquinolines) eradicate the liver forms in falciparum malaria. The liver forms in the other varieties of malaria require an 8-aminoquinoline (e.g. primaquine) to achieve eradication.

• Gametocytes may be observed in red cells for some weeks or months after cure.

MAEGRAITH (1989) p. 274

178. Vitamin D

ANSWERS: b c d

NOTES

• Vitamin D is a fat-soluble vitamin. It is also produced in the skin by action of ultraviolet light on 7-dehydrocholesterol.

• Hydroxylation, in the 25 position, occurs in the liver and the active 1,25 dihydroxycholecalciferol is produced by hydroxylation in the kidney.

• The renal hydroxylation is stimulated by parathyroid hormone, low serum phosphate and calcium. There is an alternative pathway of hydroxylation, which also occurs extrarenally, producing 24,25 dihydroxycholecalciferol. This compound has low biological activity; production is increased when serum calcium levels are high.

• 1,25 Dihydroxycholecalciferol stimulates intestinal calcium and phosphate absorption and promotes renal calcium reabsorption.

• Bone reabsorption in response to parathyroid hormone appears to occur only in the presence of active vitamin D.

DEGROOT (1995) p. 990

179. Vitamin K

ANSWERS: a c d e

NOTES

• Vitamin K is essential for hepatic synthesis of coagulation factors II, VII, IX and X.

• Vitamin K is a fat-soluble vitamin. Deficiency occurs in states of steatorrhoea (including prolonged obstructive jaundice). The vitamin is produced by the bacterial flora of the bowel, but sterilization by long-term antibiotic therapy reduces availability.

• Vitamin K crosses the placenta. However, hepatic enzymes may not be developed, especially in prematurity, and haemorrhagic disease may develop.

• When coagulation factor deficiency results from vitamin K deficiency there is an increase of factor concentrations 6–12 h after parenteral vitamin K administration.

• Coumarin anticoagulants antagonize vitamin K utilization. Their action may be reversed by the administration of large doses of vitamin K.

• The liver also synthesizes fibrinogen and possibly factor V, in addition to the vitamin K-dependent factors. The haemorrhagic tendency can usually be controlled if the levels of factors II and IX can be raised to above 30% of the normal values by transfusion of fresh frozen plasma or concentrate.

LEE *et al.* (1993) p. 570

180. Primary Sjögren's syndrome
ANSWERS: a c e

NOTES
• Sjögren's syndrome is a chronic inflammatory disorder character-ized by lymphocyte infiltration of lacrimal and salivary glands.
• Symptoms include keratoconjunctivitis sicca and xerostomia.
• Secondary cases are associated with an autoimmune disease, usually rheumatoid arthritis but less frequently SLE or systemic sclerosis.
• There is an association with renal tubular acidosis (20–40%). Proteinuria is unusual.
• Hypergammaglobulinaemia is usual and may be associated with hypergammaglobulinaemic purpura.
• Rheumatoid factor is present in most cases, as is ANF in high titre, characteristically with the speckled or nucleolar pattern of staining.
• Anti-SS-A (Ro) and anti-SS-B (La) antibodies are present in >50% of cases of primary Sjögren's syndrome but less commonly when rheumatoid arthritis is associated.
• HLA-DR3 is present in increased frequency in patients with Sjögren's syndrome. Patients with HLA-DR3 are more likely to have both SS-A and SS-B antibodies.
• There is an increased risk of lymphoma development in patients with primary Sjögren's syndrome.

KELLEY *et al.* (1993) p. 1386

181. Bilateral lower motor neuron facial palsies
ANSWERS: b c d e

NOTES
• After low motor neuron facial lesions, all forms of facial movement are lost, including that accompanying emotional expression. Upper

facial movement, preserved when the lesion is of the upper motor neuron, is paralysed when the lesion is of the lower motor neuron type. Inability to close the eye adequately may result in exposure keratitis.

• Postinfective polyneuritis (Guillain–Barré syndrome) often involves the facial nerve bilaterally. Cranial neuritis, usually in conjunction with a peripheral neuritis (polyneuritis cranialis), is associated with facial nerve palsy, usually bilateral.

• Poliomyelitis occasionally involves the brainstem, resulting in facial, pharyngeal and laryngeal paralysis.

• Uveoparotid fever (Heerfordt's syndrome), a manifestation of sarcoidosis, may be associated with facial palsy, sometimes bilateral. Infectious mononucleosis may also be a rare cause.

• Bell's palsy may, very rarely, occur bilaterally.

• Bilateral facial nerve lesions occur congenitally in the Möbius syndrome.

• Lepromatous leprosy frequently involves the facial nerve in advanced cases; this may be bilateral.

• Motor neuron disease of the midbrain predominantly affects the hypoglossal nucleus. The facial nerve may be involved but the ocular nerves are usually spared.

• Rarely cephalic tetanus may result in a lower motor neuron facial palsy.

• The facial nerves may be involved bilaterally in their intracerebral course by cerebropontine angle tumours (especially acoustic neuromas), granulomatous meningitis and leukaemic infiltration.

• The Brown-Séquard syndrome results from a hemisection of the spinal cord. It is not associated with facial nerve lesions.

• Melkersson's syndrome is associated with recurrent episodes of facial oedema and unilateral or bilateral facial palsy in patients with deeply furrowed tongues.

WALTON (1993) pp. 107, 189

182. Insulin
ANSWERS: a c d e

NOTES
• Insulin increases cell permeability to glucose; however, the liver cell appears to be permeable even under conditions of insulin deficiency and thus differs from other cells.

• Insulin stimulates glucokinase activity. This enzyme catalyses the reaction of glucose to glucose-6-phosphate.

• Insulin stimulates phosphofructokinase activity. This enzyme catalyses a further step of the glycolytic pathway. Gluconeogenesis is actively favoured when activity of this enzyme is low.

• Glycogen synthetase is stimulated by insulin. Phosphorylase, which catalyses the rate-limiting step of glycogen breakdown, is inhibited by insulin.

• In the absence of insulin, triglyceride breakdown in adipose tissue is increased and free fatty acids are released. However, hepatic free fatty acid synthesis is reduced.

• Rapid hepatic formation of triglyceride and phospholipid may continue, despite the reduced rate of glycolysis under conditions of insulin lack, when there is a flow of free fatty acids to the liver.

DEGROOT *et al.* (1995) p. 1389

183. Ulcerative colitis
ANSWERS: a b c d e

NOTES
• Colonic carcinoma associated with ulcerative colitis may result in stricture formation, but benign stricture may also occur in up to 10% of cases (usually of the sigmoid colon or rectum).

• Toxic megacolon and perforation are serious complications of fulminant disease.

• Up to 20% of cases of inflammatory bowel disease are complicated by a seronegative, often monoarticular, non-erosive arthritis. This predominantly affects the knees and ankles. Joint symptoms often accompany intestinal disease activity. Sarcoiliitis is a frequent finding in long-standing disease and is associated with iritis; occasional progression to ankylosing spondylitis occurs. Clubbing is associated, especially when the proximal colon is involved.

• Erythema nodosum and erythema multiforme are associated; pyoderma gangrenosum is almost diagnostic of ulcerative colitis and associated with active disease. Aphthous ulceration is not uncommon.

• Ophthalmic complications include iritis and episcleritis.

• Biochemical evidence of hepatic damage is common but usually asymptomatic (however, cirrhosis may occur). Pericholangitis is common but does not appear to progress to biliary cirrhosis. Primary sclerosing cholangitis is a rare complication.

SLEISENGER & FORDTRAN (1993) p. 1305

184. Juvenile rheumatoid arthritis
ANSWERS: d e

NOTES

• Juvenile rheumatoid arthritis has a peak incidence between 1 and 3 years; it is more common in girls.

• There may be a presentation with polyarthritis (40%), oligoarthritis (50%) or with a systemic illness (10%).

• In the most common oligoarticular presentation the knees are the most commonly involved joint. Extra-articular features (except uveitis) are uncommon in this form of disease. Most cases are ANA-positive.

• Chronic uveitis is particularly likely to occur in girls who have an early onset of oligoarthritis and who are ANA-seropositive. Most patients (98%) have an asymptomatic onset of uveitis.

• Inflammation and ankylosis of the posterior apophyseal joints of the upper cervical spine with atlantoaxial subluxation are characteristic of the polyarticular disease.

• In the systemic disease there is characteristically a high swinging fever and a macular, or maculopapular, rash. Generalized lymphadenopathy and splenomegaly occur. Pericarditis and pleurisy are associated.

• IgM rheumatoid factor is not usually associated (except in a minority of older children who have a polyarticular presentation); ANF is commonly present (85% of those with an oligoarticular presentation) but anti-ds DNA antibodies are not associated.

• Prognosis is best in oligoarticular and systemic features and complete remissions can be expected in 30–50% of cases

KELLEY et al. (1993) p. 1189

185. Primary hyperparathyroidism
ANSWERS: b c e

NOTES

• Excessive parathyroid hormone secretion in primary hyperparathyroidism results in bone resorption and hypercalcaemia. A single adenoma is the most common cause. Females are affected twice as often as males.

• Bone involvement ranges from subperiosteal absorption of the phalanges, resorption of the phalangeal tufts and loss of the lamina dura of the teeth, to the advanced classical, osteitis fibrosa cystica (severe demineralization, bone cysts, fractures and deformities).

• Hypercalcaemia and ectopic calcium deposition result in recurrent nephrolithiasis (although parathyroid hormone reduces renal calcium clerance), corneal calcification, chondrocalcinosis and pyrophosphate arthropathy.

• Generalized pruritis is associated. Generalized muscular weakness occurs in a minority of cases (about 5%). Behavioural and mental disturbance is common (greater than 50% of cases).

• Hyperparathyroidism may occur as part of a familial condition including:

(a) multiple endocrine adenomatosis (MEA) type I—hyperparathyroidism, pituitary adenomas and pancreatic islet cell tumours (often causing the Zollinger–Ellison syndrome)

(b) MEA type II—hyperparathyroidism, phaeochromocytoma and medullary thyroid carcinoma, Cushing's disease and carcinoid tumours

DEGROOT (1995) p. 1047

186. Diagnosis of Cushing's syndrome
ANSWERS: a b e

NOTES

• Dexamethasone (2 mg 6-hourly for 3 days) usually suppresses corticosteroid production in Cushing's disease (pituitary adenoma).

• Adenomas and carcinomas of the adrenal and ectopic ACTH-producing tumours are not usually suppressed by dexamethasone. Adenomas often produce androgens, in addition to corticosteroids. These may result in virilization and antagonism of the catabolism associated with excess glucocorticoid levels.

• 17-Hydroxysteroid excretion is affected by hepatic and renal disease; it is increased in many obese subjects. The assay reflects a significant proportion of material which does not represent cortisol metabolites.

191

- 17-Ketosteroids and 17-ketogenic steroids represent both glucocorticoid and androgenic metabolites and are thus less useful to detect glucocorticoid excess.
- Measurement of urinary free cortisol is probably the best screening test for Cushing's syndrome. A full 24-h urine collection is essential for results to be meaningful.
- ACTH levels are elevated or normal in Cushing's disease, high with ectopic ACTH production, but very low where there is an adrenal adenoma or carcinoma.

DEGROOT (1995) p. 1750

187. Hypothyroidism
ANSWERS: a b c d e

NOTES

- Thyroid-stimulating hormone (TSH) secretion increases in response to small reductions of thyroid secretion.
- TSH increases thyroid triiodothyronine secretion proportionately more than thyroxine (resulting in a higher triiodothyronine/thyroxine ratio).
- 98% of cases of hypothyroidism are primary.
- Decreased thyroid-binding globulin (TBG) or the presence of drugs which inhibit binding to TBG such as salicylate result in low thyroxine levels in the absence of hypothyroidism. Free thyroxine values are normal in those with low TBG levels.
- Most patients who are ill (but without thyroid disease) have low triiodothyronine levels.
- Determination of the TSH response to thyroid-releasing hormone is not helpful in differentiating pituitary and hypothalamic hypothyroidism, as responses are variable.

DEGROOT (1995) p. 752

188. Ulnar nerve
ANSWERS: a b c d e

NOTES

- The ulnar nerve is the main continuation of the medical cord of the branchial plexus. Fibres are derived from the eighth cervical and first

thoracic roots, with a lesser contribution from the seventh cervical.
• The nerve runs on the medial side of the artery, piercing the intermuscular sputum in the mid upper arm, to run on the posterior aspect of the medial epicondyle of the humerus. There are no branches given off in the upper arm.
• The nerve enters the forearm by passing between the heads of flexor carpi ulnaris (which it supplies) to lie on flexor degitorum profundus (the medial half of which it supplies).
• The ulnar nerve gives off dorsal and palmar cutaneous branches in the lower forearm, together with the superficial terminal branch in the hand. These nerves convey sensation from the ulnar aspect of the hand and fingers.
• The nerve enters the hand by passing over the flexor retinaculum and then divides into the superficial and deep terminal branches. The deep terminal branch innervates the hypothenar muscles, the interossei, the medial two lumbricals (sometimes the medial three) and adductor pollicis.

WALTON (1993) p. 583

189. α_1-Antitrypsin
ANSWERS: b e

NOTES
• α_1-Antitrypsin is a polymorphic glycoprotein secreted by the liver and is an important inhibitor of neutrophil elastase.
• α_1-Antitrypsin deficiency results from defective transport from hepatocytes to the blood (neonatal jaundice and infantile cirrhosis may be associated).
• Homozygotes (PiZZ) have 10% of normal levels while heterozygotes (PiMZ) have about 60%. Heterozygotes have no detectable increased risk of emphysema.
• α_1-Antitrypsin deficiency is associated with predominantly basal pulmonary emphysema. Deficiency is associated with significantly more advanced pulmonary disease in those who smoke.
• Polycythaemia and cor pulmonale are late features.
• Blood levels of α_1-antitrypsin are increased by danazol therapy or can be restored by infusion of α_1-antitrypsin concentrates.

CROFTON & DOUGLAS (1989) p. 496

190. Phenytoin
ANSWERS: b c e

NOTES
• Phenytoin is absorbed at a variable rate but is nearly totally absorbed from the gastrointestinal tract in most cases. It is 70–90% bound to plasma protein but less so in renal failure.
• Phenytoin is inactivated by the microsomal enzymes of the liver. This inactivation is inhibited by chloramphenicol, dicumarol, isoniazid and cimetidine. Concurrent therapy with these agents is associated with increased phenytoin levels.
• Phenytoin levels are reduced when carbamazepine is administered concurrently. Oral anticogulants displace phenytoin from protein binding.
• Phenytoin exerts a stabilizing effect on all neuronal membranes by blocking sodium channels and inhibits the generation of repetitive action potentials.
• Toxic effects include cerebellovestibular dysfunction, increased frequency of convulsions and behavioural abnormalities. Hirsutism and gingival hyperplasia complicate chronic administration.
• Megaloblastic anaemia is associated with chronic phenytoin therapy. It appears to result from impairment of folic acid absorption and metabolism. It responds to folic acid supplements.
• Osteomalacia is also associated with chronic administration. There appears to be both altered vitamin D metabolism and reduced gastrointestinal calcium absorption.
• A lymphadenopathy with reduced IgA production is associated with chronic therapy.

GILMAN *et al.* (1990) p.439

191. Tardive dyskinesia
ANSWER: e

NOTES
• Tardive dyskinesia is a complication which may develop after at least 6 months of chronic phenothiazine therapy. It tends to occur in older patients, especially females.
• Tardive dyskinesia is characterized by stereotypied, repetitive, involuntary movements including lip smacking, chewing and darting

movements of the tongue in and out of the mouth and choreiform movements of the limbs.

• The movements disappear during sleep, as do those of parkinsonism.

• Movements may get worse on stopping the drug or occur for the first time after discontinuation of the drug.

• Tardive dyskinesia remits in 66% of cases over the 3 years following drug withdrawal but persists in the remainder.

• Tardive dyskinesia is resistant to treatment; however high-dose anticholinergic treatment may be helpful.

• 2% of patients (who tend to be young and male) treated with phenothiazines develop dystonic reactions within hours or days of starting treatment. Intravenous anticholinergic agents abolish the movements rapidly and there is resolution on stopping the drug.

WALTON (1993) p. 349

192. Interactions of oral anticoagulants
ANSWER: a

NOTES

• Coumarins interfere with hepatic synthesis of vitamin K-dependent clotting factors (II, VII, IX, X).

• The anticoagulant action is delayed for about 36 h until the clotting factors, formed before the drug administration, have disappeared from the circulation. Oral anticoagulants cross the placenta.

• The anticoagulant activity of oral anticoagulants is antagonized by cholestyramine, which impairs gastrointestinal absorption of the drug, and by griseofulvin, barbiturates, rifampicin and glutethimide, which induce the hepatic microsomal enzymes; dangerous haemorrhage may occur when these drugs are withdrawn and oral anticoagulants continued.

• Oral anticoagulants are potentiated when vitamin K availability is reduced by low dietary intake or reduced large-bowel microflora (the colonic bacteria are an important source of vitamin K).

• Warfarin is about 97% bound to plasma protein. It is displaced from plasma protein (resulting in elevated levels of free, active drug) by phenylbutazone (which also inhibits warfarin metabolism), chloral hydrate and mefenamic acid.

• Acetylsalicylic acid impairs platelet aggregation. In patients who are taking oral anticoagulants this impairment of platelet action may be associated with significant haemorrhage. In larger doses (over 3 g/day), acetylsalicylate displaces warfarin from protein binding. Paracetamol and sodium salicylate do not interact with oral anticoagulants or affect platelet function.

• Clofibrate inhibits platelet aggregation and increases clotting factor turnover; it does not increase levels of free warfarin or inhibit warfarin metabolism. Administration of clofibrate with oral anti-coagulants may be complicated by serious haemorrhage.

• Cimetidine potentiates oral anticoagulation by an unknown mechanism. Frusemide, spironolactone, chlorpromazine and ascorbic acid have no effect on the action of oral anticoagulants.

GILMAN *et al.* (1990) p. 1319

193. *Helicobacter pylori*
ANSWER: d

NOTES
• Most cases of peptic ulceration occur in a setting of diffuse antral gastritis which is strongly associated with the presence of *Helicobacter pylori*.
• Peptic ulceration associated with non-steroidal anti-inflammatory drug use or acid hypersecretion associated with gastrinoma is not associated with antral gastritis.
• There is an increased prevalence of *H. pylori* infection with increasing age.
• 92% of patients with duodenal ulceration have *H. pylori* identified in their antral mucosa. Some 72% of patients with gastric ulcer have *H. pylori* identified.
• Gastrin release is enhanced in patients with *H. pylori*.
• Sustained eradication of *H. pylori* occurs in 20% of cases treated with bismuth but in 70% of those treated with bismuth plus tinidazole or metronidazole. Resistance to tinidazole or metronidazole seems common.
• Healing of peptic ulcers seems modestly accelerated in patients with *H. pylori* treated with bismuth tinidazole or metronidazole in addition to H_2-blocker. Rates of recurrence appear to be markedly lower in those in whom *H. pylori* is eradicated.

SLEISENGER & FORDTRAN (1993) p. 580

194. Hereditary angio-oedema

ANSWERS: a b c d e

NOTES

• Hereditary angio-oedema is due to deficiency of C1 inhibitor. It is an autosomal dominant condition with high penetrance.

• Patients are generally asymptomatic. Attacks occur in one site (usually face or one limb) and last 48–72 h. Bowel or upper respiratory tract may be involved.

• The oedema is not associated with itching, nor is it associated with urticaria.

• Trauma may provoke attacks, presumably by exhausting C1 inhibitor by activating plasmin, but most occur spontaneously.

• C1 inhibitor reacts with a variety of enzymes, including C1r, C1s, kallikrein, plasmin and coagulation factors XIIa and XIa.

• Demonstration of low levels of C1 inhibitor activity confirms the diagnosis. Most cases (90%) have low functional and antigenic C1 inhibitor levels while a minority (10%) have normal antigenic levels of dysfunctional C1 inhibitor.

• Testosterone treatment (including danazol and stanazol) enhances C1 inhibitor levels. Tranexemic acid is also effective. Both treatments may be combined.

• Attacks may be treated by replacing inhibitor using purified C1 inhibitor concentrates.

LACHMANN *et al.* (1993) p. 1293

195. Inflammatory disease of the large bowel

ANSWER: all incorrect

NOTES

• Crohn's colitis usually presents with diarrhoea and prominent colicky abdominal pain. Bloody diarrhoea is unusual. An abdominal mass may be palpated.

• In ulcerative colitis bloody diarrhoea is characteristic; while abdominal discomfort is common. Severe colicky pain is usual.

• Perianal disease (fistulae, abscesses and fissures) is more common in association with Crohn's disease. The rectum is involved in up to 50% of cases of colonic Crohn's disease, but is almost always involved in

197

ulcerative colitis (though the rectum is uninvolved by radiological criteria in about 20% of cases).

• In ulcerative colitis the inflammation is usually confined to the mucosa, but may sometimes show some spread to the submucosa. Crypt abscesses are characteristic: they may coalesce, leading to the formation of pseudopolyps. Some fibrosis and muscular hypertrophy may occur.

• The inflammation of Crohn's disease is transmural. There is more prominent fibrosis and lymphoid hyperplasia than is the case in ulcerative colitis. Granuloma formation occurs. (Crypt abscesses may also be seen in Crohn's disease.)

• Radiological evidence of ulceration and pseudopolyp formation may occur in both Crohn's and ulcerative colitis. Deep linear clefts and fistulae are characteristic of Crohn's disease.

• Segmental involvement of the left colon may occur in both Crohn's colitis and ulcerative colitis. However, segmental involvement of the transverse and right colon is almost diagnostic of Crohn's colitis. Skip lesions are diagnostic of Crohn's disease.

• Radiological abnormality of the terminal ileum often occurs in both ulcerative colitis (the so-called reflux ileitis) and in Crohn's disease of the colon.

• Narrowing of the bowel occurs in both types of inflammatory bowel disease (Crohn's and ulcerative colitis); however, eccentric narrowing is much more commonly due to Crohn's disease.

• Crohn's disease of the colon rarely appears to be complicated by the development of colonic carcinoma.

SLEISENGER & FORDTRAN (1993) pp. 1270, 1305

196. Erythrocyte sedimentation rate
ANSWERS: a b c d

NOTES

• The factors influencing the rate of sedimentation of red cells are complex; however, the degree of rouleau formation is an important factor.

• High-molecular-weight plasma proteins, especially fibrinogen, but also α_2 and gammaglobulin, increase rouleau formation and the ESR.

• Afibrinogenaemia and hypofibrinogenaemia are associated with very low rates of erythrocyte sedimentation.

- The packed cell volume (PCV) also influences the ESR. Poly-cythaemia (with a high PCV) is associated with a low ESR; anaemia is associated with a high ESR.
- Cold agglutinins result in red-cell clumping and an increased rate of precipitation, while spheroidal cells form rouleaux poorly and there-fore sedate slowly.
- Females tend to have higher levels of ESR than males, and levels tend to rise with age. High ESR results are found during pregnancy.
- C-reactive protein (which precipitates with the C-polysaccharide of the pneumococcus) concentration in the serum is elevated under similar clinical conditions to those associated with a raised ESR. The significance of C-reactive protein is unknown.

LEE *et al.* (1993) p. 30

197. IgA nephropathy
ANSWERS: a b d e

NOTES
- Mesangial proliferative glomerulonephritis with IgA deposition is one of the commonest form of glomerulonephritis in developed countries.
- There may be (in 30–35% of cases) recurrent episodes of macro-scopic haematuria (lasting 1–5 days) and often occurring 2–3 days after an upper respiratory tract infection. IgA nephropathy is the commonest form of glomerulonephritis to be associated with macro-scopic haematuria.
- In another 30–35% of cases there is proteinuria with microscopic haematuria.
- IgA nephropathy is three to six times more common in males, mainly in the second or third decade.
- IgA nephropathy is associated with alcoholic liver disease, coeliac disease and carcinomas.
- Serum IgA levels are increased in 50% of cases. Circulating IgA-containing immune complexes are commonly present in clini-cally active cases.
- Renal failure develops in 30% of cases. Sustained hypertension, persistent proteinuria and nephrotic syndrome are poor prognostic features.

SCHRIER & GOTTSCHALK (1993) pp. 1659, 1839

198. Oesophagus

ANSWER: C

NOTES

• The oesophagus is between 25 and 35 cm long. The distance from the teeth of the cardia, measured with the endoscope, is about 40 cm.
• The upper sphincter is formed by the cricopharyngeus muscle.
• The oesophagus lies in the posterior mediastinum, behind the trachea and then close to the left main bronchus. The oesophagus passes through the diaphragm behind the anterior and left tendon leaflets. The inferior vena cava passes through the central dome of the diaphragm.
• The oesophagus is lined by stratified squamous epithelium. It joins the gastric mucosa (columnar) at the ora serrata.
• The venous drainage of the lower third of the oesophagus is to the portal system by way of the gastric veins. The middle third drains to the azygous system and the upper third to the superior vena cava.
• The spinal accessory nerve (XI) carries motor fibres to the cervical oesophagus, the vagus to the remainder. The motor nerves communicate with those of Auerbach's plexus.
• The muscle fibres of the upper third of the oesophagus are striated, while those of the lower oesophagus are smooth. There is a gradual transition from one muscle type to the other.
• There is no serosal covering to the oesophagus.

SLEISENGER & FORDTRAN (1993) p. 311

199. Duodenum

ANSWERS: a b c d e

NOTES

• The duodenum is 30 cm in length. The first part (5 cm) is intraperitoneal. The bile duct and the inferior vena cava pass behind.
• The remainder of the duodenum is retroperitoneal. The second part of the duodenum runs round the head of the pancreas. The ampulla of Vater is situated in this part of the duodenum.
• The third part of the duodenum crosses over the inferior vena cava, the aorta and the origin of the inferior mesenteric artery. The superior mesenteric artery passes anteriorly.
• The fourth part of the duodenum turns upwards along the left side

of the aorta. The duodenum terminates at the ligament of Trietz, where the jejunum begins.

• There is an outer longitudinal, and an inner circular, muscle layer. Brunner's glands are most abundant in the proximal duodenum; they are not usually seen in the jejunum. The glands extend into the lamina propria. The secretion is viscous and alkaline.

• There is active mucosal iron absorption in the small bowel. Iron is then transported across the serosa. The latter step is localized to the duodenum. Calcium absorption also appears to be maximal in the duodenum.

SLEISENGER & FORDTRAN (1993) pp. 467, 793

200. Steatorrhoea
ANSWERS: c d e

NOTES

• In coeliac disease the ileum is not involved. A moderate steator-rhoea is usual (25–30 g faecal fat excretion/day). In pancreatic insufficiency a fat excretion in excess of 35 g/day is typical.

• Patients with pancreatic insufficiency tend to maintain their serum albumin levels (amino acid absorption is reasonably normal), in contrast to those with coeliac disease in whom hypoalbuminaemia is usual.

• Fat-soluble vitamin (A, D, E, K) absorption is impaired in small-bowel disease (e.g. coeliac). Symptomatic fat-soluble vitamin deficiency is uncommon in association with pancreatic disease.

• Folic acid deficiency is associated with coeliac disease and other small-bowel disorders. Folate levels are generally normal in patients with pancreatic disease, though alcohol interferes with folate metabolism.

• Vitamin B_{12} levels are typically low in Crohn's disease of the terminal ileum (the site of B_{12} absorption) and in the 'blind-loop' syndrome (where bacteria utilize intraluminal B_{12}). Levels of vitamin B_{12} are usually normal in both coeliac disease and chronic pancreatic disease. Pancreatic secretion does however appear to sensitize the B_{12} intrinsic factor complex, increasing its affinity for the receptors in the terminal ileum.

SLEISENGER & FORDTRAN (1993) pp. 1087, 2048

201. Bilirubin
ANSWERS: a c

NOTES
• Bilirubin is the product of haem metabolism. Fasting increases bilirubin production. There is almost complete binding of unconjugated bilirubin to albumin (albumin infusion in conditions of hyper-unconjugated bilirubinaemia is associated with a further increase of bilirubin levels, as bilirubin is mobilized from extracellular fluid into the circulation).
• Sulphonamides, salicylates, non-esterified fatty acids and reduced pH levels result in decreased protein binding of unconjugated bilirubin. Free unconjugated bilirubin crosses the neonatal blood–brain barrier and may result in the development of kernicterus.
• Conjugated bilirubin is also bound to albumin but less avidly than is unconjugated bilirubin.
• Bilirubin is excreted in conjugated form, mostly as a glucuronide.
• Conjugated bilirubin is not significantly reabsorbed from the gastro-intestinal tract. There is partial deconjugation and conversion of bilirubin to urobilinogen by bacteria within the bowel. Urobilinogen is reabsorbed, circulates to the liver where it is re-excreted. When the load of urobilinogen increases some may be excreted in the urine.
• Even high-concentration unconjugated bilirubin is not excreted in the urine. Conjugated bilirubin passes into the urine: this becomes an important route of excretion in obstructive jaundice.
• Bilirubin is decomposed by light, of wavelength 425–475 nm, in the visual spectrum, to soluble products which appear to be non-toxic and are rapidly excreted.

SHERLOCK & DOOLEY (1993) p. 199

202. Delayed gastric emptying
ANSWERS: a b c d e

NOTES
• There are regular gastric peristaltic contractions, at a rate of about 3/min.
• Food material in the duodenum inhibits gastric emptying. The calorific value of the food appears to be a more important determi-

202

nant of the inhibition of gastric motility than the volume (fat is thus more inhibitory than carbohydrate of protein).

• Polypeptides associated with inhibition of gastric emptying include gastrin, CCK, gastric inhibitory polypeptide and VIP. Secretin inhibits gastric motility, but does not appear to do so in physiological concentrations.

• Motilin stimulates motility and pepsin secretion (but not acid secretion). Metoclopramide stimulates gastric motility.

• Pain and bowel distension are associated with delayed gastric emptying, mediated by the autonomic nervous system. Vagotomy is associated with delayed gastric emptying, as is autonomic neuropathy such as that complicating diabetes.

• Delayed gastric emptying is associated with diabetes and may be associated with hyperglycaemia or autonomic neuropathy.

• Truncal vagotomy delays gastric emptying of solids (but this returns to normal by 3 years postsurgery). Atropic gastritis is associated with delayed emptying (in contrast to those with Zollinger–Ellison syndrome who have rapid emptying).

• Opiates and anticholinergics delay gastric emptying. Phenothiazines and H_2-receptor blockers (e.g. cimetidine) do not appear to influence gastric motility.

SLEISENGER & FORDTRAN (1993) p. 978

203. Argyll Robertson pupils
ANSWERS: a c

NOTES
• Argyll Robertson pupils are small and constant in size, unaltered by light or shade. They contract promptly on convergence and dilate again promptly when the effort to converge is relaxed.
• Argyll Robertson pupils dilate slowly and imperfectly to mydriatics.
• When the aetiology is syphilitic the pupils are typically irregular and unequal with atrophy and depigmentation of the iris and loss of the ciliospinal reflex (dilatation of the pupil when the skin of the neck on the same side is scratched with a pin).
• In congenital syphilis the pupils are often dilated and not typical of Argyll Robertson pupils.
• Rarely, Argyll Robertson pupils may occur in diabetes, alcoholic polyneuropathy and chronic hypertrophic polyneuropathy.

• In the Holmes–Adie syndrome there is moderate pupillary dilatation (unilateral in 80%) with diminished, or absent, reaction to light. There is a delayed but often excessive constriction in response to accommodation. Tendon reflexes are usually decreased or absent.
• The Marcus Gunn pupil results from a unilateral retrobulbar neuritis or neuropathy. There is a poor pupiliary reaction to light on the affacted side but the consensual reaction in that pupil to light shone in the opposite eye is brisk.

WALTON (1993) p. 90

204. Spinal cord anatomy
ANSWERS: d e

NOTES
• The spinal cord extends from the foramen magnum to the level of the lower border of the first, or the upper border of the second, lumbar vertebra. The nerve roots below this level form the cauda equina.
• The average length of the spinal cord is 45 cm.
• The spinal cord lies in the CSF within the dura, suspended laterally by the ligamentum denticulatum. The ligamentum flavum runs between adjacent vertebral laminae.
• There is an expansion of the spinal cord at the lower end, the conus medullaris, from which a fine fibrous band runs to the back of the coccyx. The dura fuses with this band (and the subarachnoid space is obliterated) at the second or third sacral vertebral level.
• The dorsal roots convey sensory fibres, the ventral roots motor. The dorsal and ventral roots remain separate until they have pierced the dura.
• The blood supply of the upper cord is derived from the two anterior spinal arteries, which are branches of the vertebral arteries. The anterior spinal arteries fuse to form a single vessel. There are also a pair of posterior spinal arteries on each side of the cord, also branches of the vertebral arteries.
• The anterior and posterior spinal arteries are reinforced along the length of the cord by radicular arteries which reach the cord via the intervertebral foramina.

WALTON (1993) pp. 23, 478

205. Chlorpromazine
ANSWER: a

NOTES

• Chlorpromazine has a sedative action and decreases spontaneous motor activity. It also has an antipsychotic action.

• Chlorpromazine blocks CNS dopamine (D_2) receptors; this results in prolactin release, antiemesis (dopamine stimulates the trigger zone) and extrapyramidal effects (due to D_1 blocking action).

• Chlorpromazine blocks adrenergic α-receptors and also has a local vasolidating action. These effects result in hypotension. Chlorpromazine also has mild anticholinergic, antihistamine and anti-5-hydroxytryptamine actions.

• Hypersensitivity reactions to chlorpromazine include blood dyscrasias and cholestatic jaundice. They usually occur within 6 weeks of the initiation of therapy.

• Dermatitis and urticaria occur in 5% of cases. Nasal stuffiness, mouth dryness and blurred vision are manifestations of the autonomic actions.

• Plasma cholesterol levels are increased in those patients on long-term chlorpromazine therapy.

• Chlorpromazine blocks the antihypertensive action of guanethidine. The sedative and miotic effects of opiates and the effects of alcohol may be potentiated.

• Chlorpromazine results in a transient increase in CSF, plasma and urine homovanillic acid excretion for about 3 weeks after initiation of treatment. Thereafter excretion is reduced.

GILMAN *et al.* (1990) p. 396

206. α-Methyldopa
ANSWERS: a b d e

NOTES

• The decarboxylation of dopa results in the formation of dopamine. This step is inhibited by α-methyl dopa. α-Methyldopa therapy is associated with reduced concentrations of dopamine, 5-hydroxytryptamine and noradrenaline in both peripheral tissues and in the CNS. Methylnoradrenaline is also produced.

- The majority hypertensive action of α-methyldopa appears to be a central action.
- α-Methyldopa therapy is associated with reduced plasma renin levels, but like most other antihypertensive drugs it tends to promote sodium and water retention. Renal blood flow is unaltered or increased.
- About 25% of the oral dose is absorbed unchanged. Most is excreted by the renal route, above 20% of the total as unchanged drug.
- Even after intravenous administration there is no hypotensive effect for 1–2 h, though a paradoxical hypertensive response may occur. The fall in blood pressure is greater in hypertensive than in normotensive individuals.
- Side-effects of α-methyldopa therapy include sedation, increased prolactin levels (sometimes with lactation), a positive Coombs antiglobulin test in 10–20% of cases (occasionally with haemolytic anaemia) and occasionally a haemolytic anaemia.
- Methyldopa treatment increases the frequency of CNS toxicity by lithium.

GILMAN *et al.* (1990) p. 789

207. Sideroblastic anaemia
ANSWERS: a b c d

NOTES
- In sideroblastic anaemia the anaemia is hypochromic and microcytic. The blood film usually shows a dimorphic picture with normochromic and hypochromic cells. There may also be anisocytosis and poikilocytosis.
- Ring sideroblasts in the bone marrow are virtually diagnostic (these are normoblasts with excessive haemosiderin deposited aroung the nuclei). Iron granules may occur in erythroblasts in thalassaemia, but ring forms are rare. There is also erythroid hyperplasia. There is raised serum iron and saturated iron-binding capacity.
- A hereditary, sex-linked, sideroblastic anaemia is rare; there is usually a response to pyridoxine (though large doses may be required).
- Primary acquired sideroblastic anaemia occurs in older adults. There is progressive anaemia and hepatosplenomegaly: eventually transfusions are required. Neutropenia and thrombocytopenia usually develop. Leucocycte alkaline phosphatase activity is usually

low. Ring sideroblasts are prominent at all stages of erythroblast maturation. Some cases may have associated folate deficiency; response to azathioprine has been reported.

• Secondary sideroblastic anaemia may complicate marrow involvement by neoplasia, collagen disease, lead poisoning, alcohol consumption and drug therapy—especially isoniazid, para-amino salicylate and cycloserine.

LEE *et al.* (1993) p. 852

208. Korsakoff's syndrome
ANSWERS: a c d

NOTES
• Korsakoff's syndrome is characterized by a gross defect of recent memory, disorientation and confabulation. Despite profound amnesia, short-term memory (digit span) is often well-preserved.
• The recollection of distant past events is almost normal.
• Pathologically, lesions are seen in the medial, dorsal pulvinar and anteroventral thalamic nuclei, mamillary bodies and terminal portions of the fornices. There is a loss of medullated fibres and nerve cells with microglial and capillary proliferation.
• Korsakoff's syndrome typically complicates chronic alcoholism.
• Thiamine deficiency is thought to be an aetiological factor in the development of Korsakoff's syndrome (including those associated with alcoholism and chronic haemodialysis).
• Korsakoff's syndrome often occurs in conjunction with Wernicke's encephalopathy. Features of Wernicke's encephalopathy include ophthalmoplegia, ataxia and disturbance of consciousness.

WALTON (1993) p. 753

209. *Mycobacterium avium* complex (MAC)
ANSWERS: c d e

NOTES
• MAC includes both *M. avium* and *M. intracellulare*.
• Although *M. avium* causes disease in birds, MAC is ubiquitous in the environment and direct contact is not required for MAC to be contracted.

• Most patients who develop MAC infection who do not have HIV infection develop pulmonary disease on a setting of previous lung disease.

• Pulmonary colonization with MAC can occur in both normal and immunosuppressed patients, so in contrast to the more virulent tuberculosis, identification of MAC in sputum does not constitute definite evidence of infection.

• Cavities associated with MAC infection tend to be smaller and with thinner walls than do those associated with tuberculosis.

• Low CD4 counts ($<100/mm^3$) are associated with development of MAC infection in AIDS patients.

• Blood cultures are highly specific for disseminated MAC infection and generally become positive within 14 days. *M. avium* is more likely to disseminate than *M. intracellulare*.

• In AIDS patients disseminated disease is characterized by fever, sweats, hepatosplenomegaly, raised alkaline phosphatase and lymph-adenopathy. Untreated disseminated MAC leads to reduced survival in AIDS patients.

• MAC is resistant to most first-line antituberculosis treatments (e.g. isoniazid and pyrazinamide) but is generally sensitive to clarithromycin or azithromycin (though resistance soon develops if monotherapy is given).

MANDELL, BENNETT & DOLIN (1995) p. 2250

210. Duchenne-type muscular dystrophy
ANSWER: b d

NOTES

• Duchenne-type muscular dystrophy is an X-linked recessive disorder. There is a high mutation rate (i.e. about 33% appear to be new mutations with no family history).

• The age of onset is usually 3–7 years. The earliest weakness is of the limb girdle muscles.

• Muscular hypertrophy, usually of the calves, is almost invariable (90%). Tendon reflexes tend to be lost in the early stages of the disease.

• There is progressive weakness leading, eventually, to respiratory insufficiency and death. Contractures and scoliosis are prominent later features. Patients are usually unable to walk by the age of 11. Death occurs during the teens or early 20s.

• Cardiac involvement appears invariable. The characteristic electro-cardiographic changes are tall R waves in the right-sided chest leads, with Q waves in the left-sided chest and limb leads. Tachycardia is common but chronic heart failure is rare.

• CK estimation on heelprick samples from newborn males is an effective method of early diagnosis.

• Serum CK estimation during adolescence has been found to be a reliable identifier of female carriers (50% of sisters of affected boys will be carriers). More accurate identification using polymerase chain reaction and gene probes is also possible.

WALTON (1993) p. 627

211. Coronary artery supply
ANSWERS: c d e

NOTES

• The right coronary artery originates from the right sinus of Valsava. It runs in the atrioventricular groove giving branches to the right ventricle. The posterior descending artery originates from the right coronary artery, at the crux cordis, in the 85% of individuals with right coronary artery dominance.

• The left coronary artery originates from the left sinus of Valsalva. The circumflex branch runs in the atrioventricular groove; the anterior descending branch runs in the anterior interventricular sulcus. The circumflex artery gives rise to the posterior descending artery in the minority of patients with left coronary artery domi-nance.

• The posterior descending artery runs in the posterior interven-tricular sulcus and supplies a posterosuperior wedge of the interven-tricular septum.

• The sinus node artery is a branch of the right coronary artery in about 60% of cases and of the left in the remainder.

• The arterioventricular node is supplied by a branch of the posterior descending artery.

• The left anterior descending artery supplies the anterior part of the left ventricle and interventricular septum, including that part in which the right bundle of His and the anterior fascicle of the left bundle are running.

• The posterior fascicle of the left bundle appears to have dual blood supply, from both the anterior and posterior descending coronary arteries.

BRAUNWALD (1992) p. 239

212. Wenckebach second-degree heart block
ANSWERS: a b c d

NOTES
• In type I (Wenckebach) second-degree heart block there is a progressive increase of the PR interval with successive beats, until a P wave is unconducted to the ventricle.
• The degree of increase of the PR interval decreases with successive beats and the RR interval thus becomes shorter with successive beats, until the longest RR interval occurs in association with the unconducted P wave.
• In type I second-degree heart block the block is usually at the level of the atrioventricular node. The QRS complexes are of normal duration (i.e. intraventricular conduction is normal) and junctional automaticity is usually unimpaired.
• In type II second-degree heart block there is sudden failure of P-wave conduction, without prior prolongation of the PR interval.
• The block is usually below the level of the atrioventricular node in type II (Mobitz) block and nearly always occurs in those with bundle branch disease. There is frequently a prolongation of the QRS complex duration. Junctional automaticity is often impaired.
• Type I block typically improves after exercise; type II block does not.
• Although type I second-degree block may progress to complete heart block (especially in older patients) this is unusual. Progression to complete heart block is frequently seen in association with type II second-degree heart block.

BRAUNWALD (1992) p. 710

213. Gonococcal arthritis
ANSWERS: b e

NOTES
• Disseminated gonococcal infection characteristically presents with polyarthritis, tenosynovitis and dermatitis.

210

• Only 25% of patients with disseminated gonococcal infection have genitourinary symptoms.
• Certain microbial characteristics (e.g. presence of pili, specific outer membrane proteins, resistance to killing by human sera *in vitro*) and patient characteristics (e.g. terminal complement deficiency C5–C9).
• Gonococcal arthritis mainly occurs in young adults
• The arthritis is polyarticular and often migratory, usually settling on one or two joints. The arthritis most often involves the knees, followed by the ankles and wrists.
• Tenosynovitis usually affects the dorsal tendon sheaths of the wrist and fingers.
• An erythematous maculopapular or vesicular rash is usual but may also be pustular, necrotic or vasculitic.
• Gonococci are rarely cultured from blood (<10%) and infrequently from synovial fluid or skin lesions (<25%). The organism can generally be cultured from the genitourinary tract.
• Patients with disseminated gonococcal infection generally become afebrile within 48 h of initiation of antibiotic treatment and joint and skin manifestations resolve shortly thereafter. Complete recovery is usual.

KELLEY *et al.* (1993) p. 1460

214. Limb-girdle muscular dystrophy
ANSWERS: b d

NOTES
• Limb-girdle muscular dystrophy has a variable age of onset, usually in the second or third decade.
• Inheritance is generally autosomal recessive, but many cases appear to result from sporadic mutation. (Rare families with autosomal dominant inheritance are recognized.)
• Initial involvement is predominantly of the shoulder girdle muscles. The pelvic girdle muscles are affected later.
• Muscular hypertrophy of the calves is not uncommon.
• Severe disability with contractures and deformity (including scoliosis) is typically present within 20 years of the onset of disease. Early death occurs in the majority of cases.
• In facioscapulohumeral muscular dystrophy the age of onset is also variable, though again it occurs most commonly in the second

decade. Inheritance is autosomal dominant (rarely recessive). Pouting of the lips and transverse smile are characteristic.

• Involvement of the face and shoulder girdle occurs first in facioscapulohumeral muscular dystrophy with elevation of the scapulae when the arms are abducted. Anterior tibial weakness is also frequent with resulting footdrop. The disease is generally associated with a normal life span.

WALTON (1993) pp. 628, 630

215. *Clostridium difficile*
ANSWERS: a b c

NOTES
• *Clostridium difficile* is found as part of the normal faecal flora in 3% of normal healthy adults and in up to 70% of neonates. It can be isolated from the stool of 10–30% of hospitalized patients; this is much more common than the occurrence of antibiotic-associated colitis (AAC).

• *C. difficile* is a spore-forming, Gram-positive, obligate anaerobe.

• *C. difficile* is the commonest cause of AAC. *Staphylococcus aureus* is an uncommon cause.

• *C. difficile* produces toxins, the most important of which are toxin A (enterotoxin) and toxin B (cytotoxin). About 25% of strains of *C. difficile* isolated from humans lack the genes responsible for toxin production and are thus non-toxigenic.

• AAC most commonly occurs in older, debilitated patients.

• Sigmoidoscopy reveals mucosal abnormality in the majority of cases, although isolated proximal colonic disease can occur.

• *C. difficile* very rarely invades the colonic tissues. Faecal white cells are observed in only 50% of cases of AAC.

• Fever, marked abdominal tenderness, peripheral blood leucocytosis and hypoalbuminaemia all suggest AAC rather than benign diarrhoea.

• AAC may occur within 24 h of starting antibiotics or up to 6 weeks after stopping antibiotics.

MANDELL, BENNETT & DOLIN (1995) p. 978

216. Farmers' lung
ANSWERS: d e

NOTES
• Farmers' lung results from inhalation to spores of the thermophilic filamentous actinomycetes bacteria to which the subject has become sensitized. *Micropolyspora faeni* or *Thermoactinomyces vulgaris* are usually incriminated.
• The organism grows in moist hay and predominantly causes symptoms when spores are liberated when the hay is moved for use, usually in winter. The condition is more prevalent in wetter regions, when harvest time is wet and when farmers are unaware of the risk.
• 3–5% of farmers have clinical symptoms but about twice as many have precipitating antibodies to the appropriate antigen.
• Farmers who smoke appear less susceptible.
• Changing to silage feeding avoids exposure to spores. Use of a respiratory filter may also help when exposure cannot be avoided.

CROFTON & DOUGLAS (1989) p. 725

217. Pulmonary embolism
ANSWERS: d e

NOTES
• In studies comparing $\dot{V}/\dot{Q}$ scanning with pulmonary angiography in suspected pulmonary embolism, embolism is confirmed angiographically in 86% of high-risk scans. But embolism has also been angiographically identified in >30% of those with low-risk scans (high false-negative rate with V/Q scanning).
• Only 70% of patients with positive lung scans have positive venograms.
• Heparin enhances the action of antithrombin III to prevent further fibrin deposition. Heparin does not enhance clot lysis.
• Patients with pulmonary embolism show more heparin resistance than do those without embolism.
• With thrombolytic treatment, while resolution of clot is more rapid, no reduction of mortality has been observed.
• Following a percutaneous Bird's nest inferior vena cava filter

213

insertion, there is a 3% incidence of recurrent pulmonary embolism and a 3% rate of inferior vena cava occlusion.

BRAUNWALD (1992) p. 1558

218. Medullary carcinoma of the thyroid
ANSWERS: a c d

NOTES

• Medullary carcinoma of the thyroid is a malignancy of parafollicular cells (these are derived embryologically from the neural crest).
• Medullary carcinoma of the thyroid may be familial, usually exhibiting a dominant pattern of inheritance (MEN II).
• In familial cases the tumour is often multifocal (within the thyroid). There is typically an early onset (before 30 years of age) and an association with phaeochromocytoma (often bilateral) and hyperparathyroidism (usually a result of parathyroid hyperplasia). There is also an association with the development of multiple mucosal neuromas.
• Medullary carcinoma of the thyroid is characteristically associated with the secretion of peptide and other biologically active substances, including calcitonin, histamine, prostaglandins and 5-hydroxytryptamine. Ectopic ACTH production is also associated.
• Basal calcitonin levels are often increased in patients with medullary carcinoma of the thyroid (usually before there is clinically detectable disease). Stimulation of calcitonin secretion may be achieved by calcium infusion in equivocal cases (alcohol and gastrin also stimulate release). High calcitonin levels can occur in other conditions and are not diagnostic of medullary carcinoma of the thyroid.
• Calcitonin is a polypeptide (32 amino acids) which appears to inhibit bone reabsorption. Although secretion is stimulated by hypercalcaemia, high levels of calcitonin are not associated with hypocalcaemia (or abnormal phosphate levels).
• Diarrhoea is associated with medullary carcinoma of the thyroid; it may result from prostaglandin or active polypeptide secretion.
• The histological examination of tumours usually reveals amyloid accumulation between the neoplastic cells.

DEGROOT (1995) p. 855

219. Innervation of the larynx

ANSWERS: a b c

NOTES

• The vocal cords are tensed by contraction of the cricothyroid muscle: this is innervated by the external branch of the superior laryngeal nerve.

• The superior laryngeal nerve is a branch of the vagus, originating from the level of the inferior vagal ganglion. The external branch innervates the cricothyroid and inferior constrictor of the pharynx; the internal branch is the main sensory nerve of the pharynx.

• The abductors and adductors of the cords are innervated by the recurrent laryngeal nerve, as is the cricopharyngeus muscle.

• Immediately after the development of a recurrent nerve lesion the cord lies close to the midline. During phonation the unaffected cord moves across the midline (to compensate). Associated cricopharyngeus paralysis results in pooling of froth in the pyriform fossa on the side of the lesion.

• If both recurrent laryngeal nerves are divided, but the superior laryngeal nerves are intact (i.e. the lesions are below the inferior vagal ganglia), then the unopposed tensors of the cords cause the cords to lie closely applied to each other (typically <2 mm separation). Stridor may occur, especially after exertion. The voice is weak but clear.

• If there is a combined lesion of both the superior and recurrent laryngeal nerves (i.e. the lesion is above the inferior vagal ganglion), then the cord assumes an intermediate 'cadaveric' position.

WALTON (1993) p. 122

220. Hepatic vein thrombosis

ANSWERS: d e

NOTES

• Obstruction of the hepatic veins results in the development of the Budd–Chiari syndrome. The site of the obstruction may be at any site from the efferent veins of the lobules to the entry of the inferior vena cava to the right atrium.

• Myeloproliferative diseases (especially PRV) are associated in 60% of cases.

• Features of the syndrome include tender hepatomegaly, abdominal pain and ascites. If total obstruction occurs, hepatic coma and death rapidly ensue.

• In chronic disease splenomegaly may develop, associated with portal hypertension. The protein content of the ascitic fluid is high (characteristic of an exudate). Hyperalbuminaemia, a prolonged PT and elevation of serum transaminases are usual features.

• Histology reveals centrilobular distension and venous pooling with haemorrhage and necrosis. Fibrosis may occur in chronic cases.

• Hepatic venous thrombosis is prone to occur in those with polycythaemia or malignant disease and those on oestrogen therapy. Tumours may also obstruct venous drainage.

• A membranous obstruction in the suprahepatic portion of the inferior vena cava is an important cause of the syndrome because it is surgically correctable.

• The syndrome may also result from multiple obstruction of the small hepatic veins (veno-occlusive disease).

• The caudate lobe has a venous drainage to the inferior vena cava separate from that of the rest of the liver. This venous drainage may avoid occlusion, in which case the caudate lobe hypertrophies (and typically takes up isotope normally or excessively during radioisotope liver scanning).

SHERLOCK & DOOLEY (1993) p. 183

221. *Pneumocystis carinii*
ANSWER: all incorrect

NOTES

• *Pneumocystis carinii* is a ubiquitous fungal organism. Some 66% of children have a titre of 1/16 or more to *P. carinii* by the age of 4.

• Immunodeficiency associated with defective T-cell function predisposes to disease due to *P. carinii*.

• Fever, cough and tachypnoea with progressive hypoxaemia are characteristic. Haemoptysis is unusual (<10%) and pleural effusion is almost unknown.

• Auscultatory signs are characteristically sparse or absent despite the diffuse changes on the chest X-ray.

• The diagnosis can be made in >50% of cases on sputum examination using Gomori methenamine-silver nitrate stain (for cysts) or

216

polychrome methylene blue or Giemsa (for trophozoites and sporozoites).

• In survivors lungs revert to normal within 6 months.

CROFTON & DOUGLAS (1989) p. 479

222. Carbon dioxide transport
ANSWERS: a b d e

NOTES

• The carbon dioxide produced in the tissues diffuses into the plasma and thence into the red cells.

• In the plasma, a small proportion of the carbon dioxide is bound to plasma proteins, forming carbamino compounds, and some reacts slowly, forming carbonic acid, which dissociates to form hydrogen ion and bicarbonate.

• A much larger proportion of the carbon dioxide enters the red cells where it is rapidly converted to carbonic acid (catabolized by carbonic anhydrase). This carbonic acid dissciates within the red cell. The resulting hydrogen ion is buffered by reduced haemoglobin, while the bicarbonate diffuses out of the cell.

• Since anionic bicarbonate is lost from the cell, electrical neutrality is maintained by a movement of chloride ions (also anions) into the cell (the chloride shift).

• About 5–10% of the total carbon dioxide carried in the venous blood is in the form of carbaminohaemoglobin (i.e. direct binding of carbon dioxide to haemoglobin). Under conditions of hypoxia, carbon dioxide binding to haemoglobin is enhanced; affinity is reduced when the haemoglobin is oxygenated.

• When haemoglobin is oxygenated in the lung there is an alteration of the tertiary structure which results in those basic side chains (e.g. the imidazole group of histidine) which buffer hydrogen ion becoming less basic. Hydrogen ion is thus liberated as the blood passes through the pulmonary circulation; this reacts with bicarbonate, reforming carbonic acid. Carbonic acid breaks down to form water and carbon dioxide, which is expired.

CROFTON & DOUGLAS (1989) p. 40

223. Granulocyte-colony stimulating factor
ANSWERS: d e

NOTES
• G-CSF is a glycoprotein. Levels are markedly increased in patients with bacteraemia.
• Neutrophil precursor cell division is enhanced by G-CSF and maturation is accelerated.
• Peak circulating neutrophil count occurs 4–6 h after intravenous and 10–12 h after subcutaneous G-CSF administration. The neutrophil counts return to baseline by 4 days.
• Neutrophil recovery after chemotherapy has been enhanced by G-CSF. Reduced rates of infection and antibiotic use have been found in treated patients.
• Idiopathic, congenital and cyclical neutropenia have also been shown to respond to G-CSF treatment.
• Granulocyte macrophage-colony stimulating factor (GM-CSF) results in increased neutrophil and monocyte counts. Eosinophil counts increase after 7 days of treatment. The presence of circulating precursor cells is also seen after GM-CSF treatment.
• Following bone marrow transplantation more rapid restoration of neutrophil numbers is seen in GM-CSF-treated patients. Infection rates are also reduced.

DEVITA, HELLMAN & ROSENBERG (1993) p. 2278

224. Oxygen affinity of haemoglobin
ANSWERS: a b d

NOTES
• Each haemoglobin molecule has four haem groups and can thus bind four oxygen molecules. When one oxygen molecule is bound structural alteration of the haemoglobin molecule results in increased oxygen affinity by the remaining haem groups.
• Each gram of haemoglobin can carry 1.39 ml of oxygen.
• High Pco_2 acidosis or raised temperature is associated with a shift of the oxygen dissociation curve to the right (lower oxygen saturation for a given Pco_2, i.e. reduced affinity). Haemoglobin then releases oxygen more readily.

• In tissues where the Po_2 is low the raised Pco_2 has a marked effect on the oxygen affinity.
• Reduced haemoglobin can bind 2,3 DPG between the β chains and the oxygen affinity is thereby much reduced (i.e. the dissociation curve is shifted to the right by 2,3 DPG).
• Red-cell 2,3 DPG synthesis is stimulated by hypoxia.
• The oxygen dissociation curve of cells containing fetal haemoglobin is well to the left of that of normal adult haemoglobin. Free fetal haemoglobin has similar affinity to adult haemoglobin. The different oxygen affinity of intact cells appears to result from the low 2,3 DPG binding by fetal haemoglobin.
• In certain rare haemoglobinopathies (e.g. haemoglobins Chesapeake, Olympia and Heathrow) oxygen affinity is increased (i.e. the oxygen dissociation curve is shifted to the left), leading to tissue hypoxia and erythrocytosis.

CROFTON & DOUGLAS (1989) p. 38

225. Down's syndrome (trisomy 21)
ANSWERS: b e

NOTES
• Congenital heart disease occurs in 40% of cases while gastrointestinal abnormalities (especially duodenal atresia and Hirschsprung's disease) are found in 5%.
• The pathological and neurochemical changes of Alzheimer's disease are present after the third decade in the brains of all individuals with Down's syndrome.
• There is a 15 times increase in the incidence of leukaemia in Down's syndrome.
• Males are infertile, while females are subfertile but capable of reproduction.
• Both the frequency of thyroid autoantibodies and hypothyroidism are increased in Down's syndrome.
• Maternal age, but not paternal age, is strongly related to the incidence of trisomy 21.
• Lower than normal maternal α-fetoprotein levels are associated with Down's syndrome.

SCRIVER et al. (1989) p. 291

226. Haematology values

NOTES
• The haemoglobin at birth is 136–196 g/l. At 3 months the normal range is 95–125 g/l, thereafter rising slowly to the adult values (male 135–180 g/l, female 115–165 g/l).
• Young red cells contain remnants of basophilic ribonucleic acid, which stains to form a reticular pattern within the cell. These cells are referred to as reticulocytes: they are slightly larger than mature cells.
• The normal reticulocyte count is below 2% of the total red-cell count. A higher proportion of reticulocytes indicates accelerated red-cell formation. Reticulocytes normally become mature red cells within 24 h; however reticulocytes persist for longer in the circulation when erythropoiesis is very active.
• The MCHC is expressed as a percentage. It is uninfluenced by cell size. The MCHC is typically normal in macrocytic anaemias and increased in hereditary spherocytosis.

LEE *et al.* (1993) p. 7

227. The proximal tubule of the nephron
ANSWERS: a b

NOTES
• In the proximal tubule of the nephron reabsorption is essentially iso-osmotic. Sodium reabsorption is an active process.
• An almost constant proportion of the filtered load is reabsorbed from the proximal tubule at different rates of glomerular filtration.
• Protein and amino acids are actively reabsorbed from the proximal tubule.
• There is active glucose reabsorption from the proximal tubule. This active transport mechanism for glucose is saturated when the blood glucose level reaches about 10 mmol/l and glucose then appears in the urine. When the GFR is low, then higher levels of intraluminal glucose may be reabsorbed and no glycosuria occurs despite high blood glucose levels.
• There is titratable acid and ammonium ion secretion from the tubular cells, with net bicarbonate reabsorption. The active acid-

secreting mechanism also transports penicillins, probenecid and para-aminohippurate.

• Under most physiological conditions almost all of the filtered potassium delivered to the proximal tubule is reabsorbed.

SCHRIER & GOTTSCHALK (1993) p. 15

228. Oral lesions in skin disease
ANSWERS: a c

NOTES

• Pemphigus vulgaris is characterized by flaccid intraepidermal bullae, occurring on otherwise normal-looking skin. Oral lesions are usual at presentation; otherwise the oral mucosa almost invariably becomes involved as the disease progresses.

• Oral lesions occur in 20% of cases of pemphigoid, usually as a late feature.

• Dermatitis herpetiformis is associated with erythematous, vesicular or bullous lesions, with intense pruritis. Any region of skin may be involved; mucous membranes are rarely affected.

• Lichen planus is often associated with involvement of the buccal mucous membrane (in up to 70% of cases).

• Recurrent orogenital ulceration is a prominent feature of Behçet's syndrome.

• Erythema multiforme is associated with oral lesions in about 40% of cases, though involvement is usually mild. Oral lesions are a constant and severe feature of the Stevens–Johnson syndrome.

• Mucous membrane involvement in psoriasis is very rare. It is not a feature of pityriasis rosea.

CHAMPION *et al.* (1992) p. 2709

229. Lung function in asthma
ANSWERS: a c e

NOTES

• The diameter of the airways is smaller during expiration: airways obstruction is thus more profound during expiration.

• The forced vital capacity (FVC) is of similar volume to the vital capacity (VC), unless there is significant air trapping (as occurs in obstructive airways disease). During attacks patients breathe at higher lung volumes (with increased residual volume). Large negative pressures are required to achieve adequate tidal volume.

• During an asthmatic attack both the FVC and the forced expiratory volume in unit time (e.g. FEV_1) are reduced. However the FEV_1 is more reduced than the FVC, the ratio between the two values typically being below 70% (normally about 80%).

• The functional residual capacity (FRC) is the volume of gas remaining in the lung after quiet expiration. This and the residual volume (RV), which is the volume of gas remaining after maximal voluntary expiration, are usually increased during asthmatic attacks. Respiration therefore occurs with the lungs in a more inflated stage than is normal; as a consequence, the inspiratory capacity is reduced.

• The total lung capacity (TLC) is the sum of the VC and the RV: it is unaltered or increased in asthma. The VC normally constitutes about 80% of the TLC. As the RV is usually increased in asthma, the VC will be reduced.

• Static compliance reflects the elasticity of the lungs. Dynamic compliance (i.e. compliance during respiration) is influenced by airways obstruction.

• Hypoxia (a reduced arterial Pao_2) is usual during a moderately severe attack of asthma. The $Paco_2$ is typically normal or reduced, unless the attack is severe, when both a respiratory acidosis and metabolic acidosis (due to tissue hypoxia) may occur.

CROFTON & DOUGLAS (1989) p. 688

230. Sexual precocity
ANSWER: a

NOTES

• Sexual precocity is 'constitutional' in about 80% of cases in girls and 50% in boys. Some cases show familial pattern.

• In the constitutional form of precocious puberty there is normal gonadotrophin release and ovulation. The normal sequence of development with breast (thelarche) and pubic hair (pubarche) growth preceding menses (menarche) is maintained.

• Tumours of the hypothalamic region, internal hydrocephalus, encephalitis, meningitis and cerebral trauma may be associated with premature gonadotrophin release and precocious puberty.

- In the McCune–Albright syndrome precocity may occur in association with polyostotic fibrous dysplasia and patchy skin pigmentation. Gonadotrophin levels are elevated.
- Oestrogen-secreting tumours of the ovary (granulosa cell) may induce premature menstruation. Gonadotrophin levels are low and cyclical menstruation does not occur.
- Adrenal tumours may be associated with pubic hair development but menstruation is unusual.
- Congenital adrenal hyperplasia, due to 21β-hydroxylase deficiency, is associated with hirsutism and phallic hypertrophy in boys, and with hirsutism and lack of sexual development in girls.
- Patients with precocious puberty tend to be taller than their peers; however, premature fusion of the epiphyses occurs, resulting in early cessation of growth. The height of patients thus falls below that of normal individuals by the time adulthood is reached.
- Hypothyroidism is associated with precocious puberty.

HART (1985) p. 695

231. Acute leukaemia (prognostic factors)
ANSWERS: a b d e

NOTES
- Two-thirds of adults with AML have cytogenetic abnormalities.
- In AML, patients with the cytogenetic abnormality $t(8;21)$ or $inv(16)$ have an excellent response to therapy with a >90% complete remission rate and 30–40% long-term survival—in contrast to those who are diploid (no abnormality), who have a 70% chance of remission and 20% long-term remission.
- Patients with AML who have lost all or part of chromosome 5 or 7 or have an additional chromosome 8 have a low remission rate (<50%) with few (<5%) attaining long-term remission. These abnormalities are more common in patients with secondary AML complicating myelodysplastic syndrome.
- Preceding myelodysplastic syndrome is an adverse prognostic factor in AML.
- Patients with B-cell ALL have a lower complete remission rate while those with T-cell ALL have a better prognosis.
- Adults with ALL who have diploid (normal karyotype) cells have a better remission rate than do those with cytogenetic abnormality.

Hyperdiploidy (>50 chromosomes) is common in good-prognosis childhood ALL, but is rare (<5%) in adults.
• All patients with the Philadelphia chromosome eventually relapse.

DEVITA, HELLMAN & ROSENBERG (1993) pp. 1946, 1957

232. Bacteria in the bowel
ANSWERS: c d e

NOTES
• The normal small bowel contains between 10^3 and 10^5 bacteria per millilitre. In the upper small intestine streptococci, staphylococci, lactobacilli and fungi predominate. The flora of the lower small intestine more closely resembles that of the large bowel, mainly *Bacteroides* and bifidobacteria, but also lactobacillus and streptococci.
• Should the bowel mobility be reduced (as in the blind-loop syndrome), then bacterial proliferation proceeds. Intestinal hydrolysis of conjugated bile salts is increased. Free salts are unable to form micelles with dietary fat (so steatorrhoea occurs) and have a toxic action on the bowel wall.
• The bacteria liberate vitamin B_{12} from intrinsic factor and compete with the patient for this vitamin. Megaloblastic anaemia may develop. Folic acid is produced by intestinal bacteria and levels are usually high in association with bacterial proliferation.
• Indole is formed by intestinal bacteria from tryptophan; it is absorbed and excreted in the urine. The quantity excreted gives a measure of intestinal bacterial numbers.
• Radiocarbon-labelled glycocholic acid may be given orally. It is deconjugated by the bacteria. The glycine thus produced is metabolized and labelled carbon dioxide is exhaled. This gives an index of intestinal bacterial activity.
• Intestinal organisms, especially those in the colon, produce urease which decomposes the urea, diffusing into the bowel to form ammonia which is reabsorbed. Most of the ammonia produced in the body is produced in the colon.
• This ammonia production may be limited by purgation and by antibiotic therapy (e.g. neomycin). This is important in liver failure.

SLEISENGER & FORDTRAN (1993) p. 1106

233. Wilson's disease
ANSWERS: b c d

NOTES

• Wilson's disease is characterized by hepatic cirrhosis, degeneration of the basal ganglia and greenish-brown pigmented rings in the periphery of the cornea (Kayser–Fleischer rings).

• Inheritance is autosomal recessive.

• Kayser–Fleischer rings can be absent in up to 30% of cases presenting acutely with liver disease.

• Caeruloplasmin levels are low but may increase with an acute-phase response. Caeruloplasmin levels do not correlate with disease severity.

• Serum copper levels are almost invariably low but may be high in the presence of massive copper release from hepatocytes during fulminant hepatitis. Urinary copper excretion is increased.

• Liver copper levels are much increased. There is reduced biliary copper excretion with increased urinary copper excretion. Associated renal tubular damage is common.

• Penicillamine is the treatment of choice and must be continued in high dose for a long time (>2 years) before failure is accepted or copper stores are depleted. Albumin binds copper and may be useful in acute situations, as may plasmapheresis. Neurological disease carries a poor prognosis for improvement.

• Indian childhood cirrhosis is also associated with very high hepatic copper levels (>1000 µg/g).

SHERLOCK & DOOLEY (1993) p. 400

234. Acetylcholine
ANSWERS: a d e

NOTES

• Acetylcholine is the transmitter at the neuroeffector junction of all postganglionic parasympathetic fibres.

• Sympathetic vasodilator fibres to blood vessels are cholinergic (these vessels dilate as part of the anticipatory response to exercise), as are those sympathetic fibres which stimulate sweating.

• The neurotransmitter at all autonomic ganglia (both sympathetic and parasympathetic) is acetylcholine. Acetylcholine is also released

by the sympathetic nerves in the adrenal medulla, resulting in adrenaline release.
• Acetylcholine is the transmitter at the neuromuscular junction.
• Acetylcholine is rapidly hydrolysed by cholinesterase to choline and acetic acid, both of which are inactive as neurotransmitters. There is significant reuptake of acetylcholine into nerve endings; however, choline is actively reabsorbed.
• Catechol O-methyltransferase catalyses the methylation of noradrenaline and adrenaline.

WALTON (1993) p. 9

235. Antidiuretic hormone release
ANSWERS: d e

NOTES
• Throughout the body there is free movement of water across cellular membranes, governed only by the forces of osmosis and diffusion. The osmolality of intracellular and extracellular fluid thus remains similar (285–290 mosmol/l).
• The only site where free movement of water is inhibited is in the distal nephron of the kidney; here ADH increases the permeability.
• The supraorbital part of the hypothalamus appears to be the site of central control of ADH secretion, which occurs from the posterior pituitary.
• ADH secretion occurs in response to cellular dehydration, hypotension (mediated by baroreceptor afferents), decreased tension in the great veins, emotional stress, pain and raised temperature at the hypothalamus.
• Angiotensin potentiates ADH release, as do certain drugs including cholinergics, morphine, barbiturates and nicotine.
• Alcohol is a potent inhibitor of ADH secretion.
• Plasma infusion expands the intravascular volume and distends the great veins, inhibiting ADH release.

DEGROOT et al. (1995) p. 411

236. *Toxoplasma gondii*

ANSWERS: c e

NOTES

• *Toxoplasma gondii* is a sporozoon organism of the order Coccidia, suborder Eucoccidia. The trophozoite can only multiply within cells. Cells of the reticuloendothelial system are predominantly affected.

• *Toxoplasma* is transmitted to humans by ingestion of tissue cysts in raw or undercooked meat. Lamb and pork are commonly infected (up to 25% of samples).

• When immunity develops cysts form, especially in the eye, brain and skeletal muscle. Slow multiplication proceeds and cysts expand.

• *Toxoplasma* infection during pregnancy (in those without previous immunity) is associated with congenital infection. This may take the form of systemic infection (with hepatosplenomegaly), neurological deficit (often associated with calcification in the ependymal region of the lateral ventricles) or chorioretinitis or a combination of features. A markedly raised CSF protein is a hallmark of congenital toxoplasmosis.

• Multifocal encephalitis with vasculitis and necrosis may occur, particularly where toxoplasmosis complicates AIDS. Ring enhancement is characteristic of the lesions on contrast CT scanning (double-dose delayed scanning may improve the diagnostic rate).

• Ophthalmic involvement by toxoplasmosis is characteristically associated with choroidoretinitis.

• <20% of *Toxoplasma* infections in the adult are asymptomatic. Commonly there is lymphadenopathy, together with fever and non-specific symptoms.

• Acute toxoplasmosis is diagnosed by the isolation of *Toxoplasma* from blood or body fluids or by the identification of trophozoites in tissue samples. Serological tests are the primary method of diagnosis; however, antibodies are present in a high proportion of the population and may persist at high concentration for years, and this may complicate interpretation.

• A skin test is available but does not become positive until about 2 months after infection. This is useful for population surveys since false-positives are rare.

• Treatment is rarely required in immunocompetent patients. Pyrimethamine and sulphonamide are effective in those with complications and in immunocompromised patients. Trimethoprim–

sulphamethoxazole has proved to be ineffective. Treatment of pregnant women with acute infection reduces the incidence of congenital infection.

MANDELL, DOUGLAS & BENNETT (1990) p. 2090

237. Stimulants of gastrin secretion
ANSWERS: b d e

NOTES
• The cephalic phase of gastric acid secretion is mediated by the vagus. Vagal activity directly stimulates oxyntic cell acid production, but also appears to promote gastrin release (this release is markedly enhanced by prior atropine treatment).
• Acetylcholine, gastrin, histamine and calcium all stimulate oxyntic cell acid secretion.
• Gastrin is present in greatest concentration in the gastric antrum. Release is mainly stimulated by peptides and amino acids in the lumen. Glucose and fat in the stomach may be associated with a slight rise in the circulating gastrin concentration; however, acid secretion is not increased.
• Gastric distension results in vagal stimulation and some gastrin release (this release is markedly enhanced by prior atropine treatment).
• Duodenal peptide or amino acid perfusion is associated with gastrin production. The gastric acid output which results is greater than anticipated from the gastrin concentration: a second hormone which also stimulates acid secretion is postulated.
• Massive small-bowel resection is sometimes associated with hyper-gastrinaemia and acid hypersecretion. Deficiency of an inhibitory hormone is postulated.
• Acid in the gastric antrum (pH <3) inhibits gastrin release. However, antacids (in the absence of food) do not stimulate gastrin release.
• Vagotomy markedly reduces basal acid secretion and that in response to histamine or pentagastrin (a synthetic analogue of gastrin). The acid secretion normally induced by glucopenia is absent or markedly reduced after vagotomy; this is the basis of the insulin test.

SLEISENGER & FORDTRAN (1993) pp. 31, 526

238. Characteristics of lymphocytes
ANSWERS: b c

NOTES
• B lymphocytes are associated with the development of humoral immunity.
• B lymphocytes are bursa-dependent—that is to say, they become depleted if the bursa of Fabricius is excised from chicks. There is no bursa of Fabricius in humans and B lymphocytes appear to be produced in the haemopoietic tissue.
• The major B-cell population comprises newly formed small B cells which express surface IgM and IgD. These cells are poised to proliferate and produce antibody in response to antigenic stimulation.
• B cells are the predominant cell type in the primary germinal follicles of lymph nodes.
• T lymphocytes are thymus-dependent: they are associated with cell-mediated immunity. Some subsets of T cells also facilitate antibody production by B cells, while other T cells inhibit specific antibody production: these are termed helper and suppressor cells respectively.
• About 75% of the circulating lymphocytes are of the T cell type. T cells appear to be long-lived (months) and are the predominant cell found in the paracortical region of lymph nodes.

LACHMANN et al. (1993) pp. 433, 447

239. Syphilis serology
ANSWERS: b d

NOTES
• Reagin tests for syphilis use a non-treponemal antigen (cardiolipin-cholesterol-lecithin), a purified preparation of which is used in the Venereal Disease Research Laboratory (VDRL) test.
• The VDRL (the rapid plasma reagin (RPR) and automated reagin test (ART) are similar) becomes negative after treatment of syphilis and can be used to assess the effectiveness of treatment. The VDRL only becomes negative 1 year after effective treatment of primary syphilis and 2 years after treatment of secondary syphilis.
• Transient false-positive reactions to reagin tests occur in association

with infections (malaria, tuberculosis, leprosy, leptospirosis and infectious mononucleosis). They may also occur during pregnancy. Increased rates also occur with advancing age (false-positivity up to 10% of those aged >70 years). Prolonged false positivity may occur in association with SLE and rheumatoid disease.

• In the specific tests the antigen employed is treponemal material. The *Treponema pallidum* haemagglutination test (TPHA) is an example of a standard specific test. These tests do not revert to negative despite treatment.

• The most specific test is the *T. pallidum* immobilization test (TPI) but it is expensive and rarely used.

• Other spirochaetal illnesses, such as leptospirosis, yaws and rat-bite fever (*Spirillum minor*) also give positive VDRL and TPHA tests. *Borrelia burgdorferi* infection (Lyme disease) gives a positive TPHA but negative VDRL.

MANDELL, BENNETT & DOLIN (1995) p. 1803

240. *Haemophilus influenzae*
ANSWER: ALL INCORRECT

NOTES
• *Haemophilus influenzae* is a small Gram-negative bacillus. It is non-motile and non-sporing. The organism has a specific requirement for haemin (factor X) and for nicotinamide-adenine dinucleotide (factor V). *S. aureus* produces factor V: colonies of *H. influenzae* grow more avidly in the region of staphylococcal colonies as a result—this is referred to as satellitism.

• Chocolate agar (heated blood agar) provides abundant quantities of both factor V and factor X. Culture on this medium is associated with a good growth of *H. influenzae*.

• Many healthy individuals (60%) carry non-capsulate strains of *H. influenzae* in their nasopharynx. These non-capsulate strains are associated with bronchial infection in those with acute exacerbations of chronic bronchitis and with bronchiectasis.

• A smaller proportion of healthy individuals carry capsulate strains of *H. influenzae* in their nasopharynx. There are six capsulate types (a–f). Capsulate strains of *H. influenzae* are associated with meningitis, acute epiglottitis and lobar pneumonia (especially type b).

• Sensitivity to Optochin (ethyl hydrocuprein hydrochloride) is a feature of pneumococci which distinguishes them from *Streptotoccus viridans* (both produce α-haemolysis when cultured on blood agar).

CROFTON & DOUGLAS (1989) p. 321

241. Antiglomerular basement membrane antibody-mediated nephritis (Goodpasture's disease)
ANSWERS: c e

NOTES
• Antiglomerular basement disease is associated with HLA-DR2 or HLA-DR4 in 94% of cases.
• Rapid progression of renal disease to renal failure is usual and does not subsequently improve with treatment.
• Pulmonary haemorrhage is associated in most cases (which may remain alveolar and be unassociated with haemoptysis). Smoking appears to predispose to pulmonary haemorrhage.
• Pulmonary disease may occur first in the presence of normal renal function which subsequently deteriorates (sometimes up to 1 year later).
• Anaemia (frequently with features of iron deficiency) is out of proportion to that anticipated by the degree of renal failure as a consequence of pulmonary sequestration of blood.
• Linear binding of IgG to the basement membrane is almost diagnostic of antiglomerular basement disease, especially in the presence of crescentic glomerulonephritis.
• Antiglomerular basement membrane antibody is most reliably measured using an immunoassay. Once antibody levels are reduced to normal levels (usually within 1 year), recurrence is unusual.

SCHRIER & GOTTSCHALK (1993) p. 1865

242. Anterior internuclear ophthalmoplegia
ANSWER: e

NOTES
• In anterior internuclear ophthalmoplegia there is dissociation of conjugate lateral eye movement (Harris's sign).
• There is usually weakness of medial rectus movement (adduction) with normal lateral rectus movement on lateral gaze. However,

medial movement is normal when the eyes converge (may be unilateral or bilateral).

• Phasic nystagmus occurs only in the abducting eye.

• The pathological lesion is thought to be of the ascending fibres of the medial longitudinal fasciculus. The medial longitudinal fascicular fibres link the oculomotor nuclei. Multiple sclerosis is almost invariably the cause (rarely tumour or infarction).

• The fibres ascending in the posterior column of the spinal cord synapse in the gracilis and cuneatus nuclei in the posterior medulla. The fibres then decussate and ascend in the medial lemniscus.

WALTON (1993) p. 95

243. Hypertrophic obstructive cardiomyopathy
ANSWERS: a e

NOTES

• HOCM often appears as a familial condition, being inherited as an autosomal dominant condition (with a high degree of penetrance).

• There is disproportionate hypertrophy of the interventricular septum with respect to the free left ventricular wall. There is disorganization of the fibres within the hypertrophied muscle (however, this is not pathognomonic of HOCM).

• The compliance of the hypertrophied ventricle is reduced, the left ventricular end-diastolic pressure is thus elevated and the atria dilated or hypertrophied.

• The obstruction to left ventricular outflow develops as the ventricle contracts. The initial rate of ejection is normal (i.e. the initial upstroke of the carotid pulse is normal). Obstruction then occurs, finally followed by a further phase of ejection. Obstruction to outflow is associated with an abnormal movement of the anterior mitral valve leaflet toward the ventricular septum (identifiable on echocardiography).

• Features on examination include left ventricular lift, loud third and fourth sounds and a harsh late systolic murmur (due to turbulence as the blood passes the outflow obstruction or due to the mitral regurgitation which invariably accompanies the obstruction). The murmur does not tend to radiate into the neck, in contrast to that associated with aortic valve stenosis.

• Atrial fibrillation may occur and often results in a marked clinical deterioration (since the atrial contraction is an important factor maintaining ventricular filling against the resistance of the hypertrophied ventricle). Bacterial endocarditis may occur–prophylaxis is indicated.

• Electrocardiographic ST and T-wave abnormalities are common. Prominent Q waves, especially in the inferior and left-sided leads, are frequent.

• The magnitude of obstruction (and hence the clinical features) is increased if the ventricular volume is low. Stimulation of myocardial contraction (e.g. by isoprenaline or digoxin), a reduced preload (e.g. as follows the Valsalva manoeuvre) or a reduced afterload (e.g. by amyl nitrate or nitroglycerin administration) all increase the degree of obstruction.

• β-Adrenergic blockade or verapamil therapy reduces the degree of obstruction (or prevents the increase associated with exercise). Surgical excision of a portion of the obstruction muscle may be beneficial.

BRAUNWALD (1992) p. 1404

244. Coagulation tests
ANSWER: a

NOTES

• The PT is an approximate measure of the extrinsic coagulation pathway. Tissue thromboplastin is provided by brain or lung extract and kaolin is present to ensure contact activation. The PT is influenced by the levels of prothrombin (factor II) and factors V, VII and X. Heparin therapy and hypofibrinogenaemia are also associated with a prolongation of the PT.

• The PTT is an approximate measure of the intrinsic coagulation pathway. Phospholipid (e.g. cephalin) is used to replace platelet activity in the test. The test is influenced by levels of factors XII, XI, IX, VIII and, less so, factors X and V.

• Factors XI and XII are artificially activated by kaolin in the partial thromboplastin test. Unless there is a gross abnormality of these factors, the test will be unaffected.

• The thrombin time measures the rate of conversion of fibrinogen to fibrin when thrombin has been introduced. The test is abnormal in the presence of heparin and in association with disseminated intravascular coagulation.

233

- The bleeding time is influenced by the vascular response (vasospasm) and by the development of a platelet 'plug'. The results are variable when the test is repeated in the same individual.
- The tourniquet (Hess) test is performed by raising the intracapillary pressure by occluding venous drainage with a tourniquet. In a positive test petechiae develop; this is usually associated with thrombocytopenia but may occur in normal individuals.

LEE *et al.* (1993) p. 1310

245. Extrinsic allergic alveolitis (hypersensitivity pneumonitis)
ANSWER: C

NOTES
- Extrinsic allergic alveolitis is basically the result of type III allergic reaction to inhaled antigen. It develops in non-atopic individuals after prolonged exposure to certain antigens.
- Acute symptoms typically occur 5–6 h after exposure to antigen. There is cough and dyspnoea with fever, malaise and generalized aches and pains. In other cases there are no acute features, but insidious development of chronic fibrotic lung disease. In these cases the association with the antigen is less obvious.
- On auscultation during the acute phase fine crepitations may be heard. There is no wheeze.
- In acute cases the chest X-ray may show diffuse micronodular shadowing. Radiological features of chronic cases include fibrosis and a honeycomb appearance, usually most marked in the upper zones.
- The defect on lung function testing is restrictive with impaired gas transfer.
- Precipitins to the sensitizing antigen may be present. Eosinophilia is not a feature.
- Farmers' lung is the most frequently encountered form of extrinsic allergic alveolitis in the UK. The antigens are spores of thermophilic actinomycetes (especially *Micropolyspora faeni*). Precipitins to farmers' lung hay (FLH) antigen are present in 80% of cases; however about 18% of individuals with precipitins have no evidence of disease.

CROFTON & DOUGLAS (1989) p. 715

246. Haemochromatosis
ANSWERS: b d e

NOTES

• Haemochromatosis is characterized by increased absorption of dietary iron, and iron deposition. Inheritance is autosomal dominant; however, the majority of cases appear to rise sporadically.

• The condition is much more commonly seen in males. Presentation is usually in the third to sixth decade.

• Right upper quadrant abdominal discomfort is common. Hepatomegaly is a feature, but hepatocellular failure, ascites and portal hypertension are rare, late features.

• The triad of cirrhosis, diabetes (due to pancreatic iron deposition) and a slate-grey skin pigmentation are characteristic. Clinical diabetes occurs in two-thirds of cases.

• Other features include:

(a) anterior pituitary failure

(b) testicular atrophy

(c) congestive cardiac failure

(d) arthropathy (chondrocalcinosis and pyrophosphate arthropathy).

• The development of hepatocellular carcinoma is a risk and occurs in 14% of cases.

• Serum iron levels are increased; iron-binding capacity is more saturated (90%) than normal (30%). Ferritin levels are generally raised and correlate with body iron stores. Haemoglobin, white cell and platelet counts are normal.

• Desferrioxamine chelates iron and may be employed therapeutically; however, venesection is the usual choice of treatment (10 ml of blood contains about 5 mg of iron). An effective low-iron diet is impossible to achieve.

SHERLOCK & DOOLEY (1993) p. 390

247. Sarcoidosis
ANSWERS: a c e

NOTES

• Sarcoidosis is a mutltisystem granulomatous disorder of unknown aetiology. The epithelioid cell granulomas do not caseate.

• Bilateral symmetrical hilar lymphadenopathy is the most common manifestation of acute disease. Erythema, often with a polyarthritis, may be associated.

• 80% of cases of hilar lymphadenopathy due to sarcoidosis resolve within a year (90% within 2 years). In a minority parenchymal lung involvement and other features of chronic disease become apparent.

• When parenchymal lung disease develops, the symptoms associated are usually minor in relation to the radiological abnormality. Most cases spontaneously resolve; steroid therapy increases this proportion.

• Clubbing is not a feature of sarcoid lung disease.

• Features of chronic sarcoidosis include pulmonary fibrosis, uveitis, lupus pernio, peripheral neuropathy, meningoencephalopathy, hypercalcaemia, hypercalciuria and bone cysts. Splenomegaly is common.

• Uveoparotid fever (Heerfordt's syndrome) is a rare manifestation of sarcoidosis. Features include uveitis, parotid swelling and facial palsy.

• Hypergammaglobulinaemia is common in sarcoidosis: serum ACE levels tend to be raised. The delayed hypersensitivity reaction is decreased in sarcoidosis (e.g. the reaction to intradermal tuberculin or *Candida albicans*). The Kveim test is positive in 75% of those with active disease. ACE levels are increased in 75% of cases of acute sarcoidosis (also raised in Gaucher's disease, leprosy and atypical myobacterial infections).

• Decreased pulmonary gas transfer is the earliest abnormality to be detected on lung function testing. An abnormal measurement often precedes detectable radiological abnormality.

CROFTON & DOUGLAS (1989) p. 630

248. Segmental demyelination of peripheral nerves
ANSWERS: d e

NOTES
• Nerve conduction studies in cases of demyelination include a marked delay of the nerve conduction velocity and reduced amplitude of evoked action potentials.

• Nerve conduction velocity in cases of axonal degeneration is generally little delayed until the late stage of complete nerve failure.

• Electromyography in cases of axonal degeneration typically shows fibrillation potentials (which may also occur in patients with primary myopathies) and loss of motor units with reduced interference pattern. There may be evidence of reinnervation with polyphasic action potentials of increased amplitude and duration.

• In demyelination the EMG usually reveals little abnormality apart from some increased interference.

• Most neuropathies have elements of both demyelination and axonal degeneration. The defect is predominantly demyelination in lead poisoning, diphtheric neuropathy, postinfectious polyneuropathy, diabetes mellitus and leprosy.

• Predominant axonal degeneration occurs in motor neuron disease, poliomyelitis, nerve ischaemia, uraemia, in attacks of acute intermittent porphyria and as a result of damage from toxins (including drugs).

WALTON (1993) p. 358

249. Juxtaductal aortic coarctation
ANSWERS: b c d

NOTES

• Coarctation of the aorta occurs most commonly in the juxtaductal region, usually just below the origin of the left subclavian artery.

• There appears to be an association with decreased aortic and increased ductus arteriosus blood flow during intrauterine development.

• Reduced aortic blood flow occurs in cases of bicuspid aortic valve and ventricular septal defect, both of which are associated with coarctation.

• Conditions associated with augmented intrauterine aortic blood flow (e.g. pulmonary valve stenosis and tetralogy of Fallot) are almost never associated with coarctation of the aorta.

• Coarctation of the aorta occurs much more commonly in males than in females (two to five times as commonly); there is an association with Turner's syndrome. Aortic coarctation is not associated with the Noonan syndrome.

• Coarctation may lead to left ventricular failure during infancy. Those surviving 2 years usually remain asymptomatic until the second or third decade.

• Complications include those of hypertension, which occurs in the area of the arterial supply above the coarctation. Berry aneurysms of the circle of Willis are more frequently seen than in the general

population: subarachnoid haemorrhage is a well-recognized complication. Bacterial infection may develop at the coarctation or on an
associated biscuspid aortic valve. Antibiotic prophylaxis is indicated.
• Examination usually reveals hypertension in the upper limbs, with
reduced pressure in the lower. Radiofemoral delay is characteristic.
There may be a systolic murmur, sometimes lasting into diastole: it
typically radiates widely over the precordium and back. Bruits may
also be heard over collateral vessels.
• The enlarged collateral vessels may lead to notching of the ribs
which can be seen on the chest X-ray: this is not apparent before 4
years of age. The double aortic knuckle may also be seen on X-ray.

BRAUNWALD (1992) p. 920

250. Bilateral diaphragmatic paralysis
ANSWERS: a c d e

NOTES
• Bilateral diaphragmatic paralysis is associated with a decreased
maximal inspiratory force, but a normal maximal expiratory force
• VC is reduced.
• Dyspnoea, which is exacerbated by lying down, is a usual feature.
Hypoxia is also exacerbated by lying down and results from increased
ventilation–perfusion inequality.
• There is characteristically increased respiratory difficulty when the
patient is immersed in water since the diaphragms are pushed up into
the thorax by the hydrostatic pressure on the abdomen.

CROFTON & DOUGLAS (1989) p. 1168

251. Angiotensin-converting enzyme inhibitor therapy
ANSWERS: d e

NOTES
• ACE inhibitors result in reduced angiotensin I levels and markedly
increased plasma renin levels.
• Bradykinin metabolism is inhibited by ACE inhibition and levels are
consequently increased.
• Results in reduced angiotensin I levels and markedly increased
plasma renin levels.

• Bradykinin metabolism is inhibited by ACE inhibition and levels are consequently increased.
• Catecholamine levels are reduced following ACE inhibitor treatment.
• ACE inhibition is effective in heart failure regardless of the pretreatment level of plasma renin. There are actions on both arteriolar and venous beds.
• Reduced symptoms, improved exercise tolerance, reduced cardiac diameter and mortality have all been recognized in clinical trials of ACE inhibitors.

BRAUNWALD (1992) p. 496

252. *Torsade de pointes*
ANSWERS: a b c e

NOTES
• *Torsade de pointes* is a specific type of ventricular tachycardia characterized by QRS complexes of changing amplitude which appear to twist around the isoelectric line at a rate of 200–250/min.
• There is an association with a long QT interval and/or polymorphic U waves on the ECG prior to the onset of the tachycardia.
• Precipitants include bradycardia (including complete heart block), hypokalaemia, class IA antiarrhythmic drugs (quinidine, disopyramide, procainamide) and possibly classes IC and III also.
• Class IB drugs (e.g. lignocaine, phenytoin) do not prolong the QT interval and may be effective treatment. β-Blockade is the preferred treatment. Magnesium infusion or pacing may also be effective.

BRAUNWALD (1992) p. 708

253. Somatostatin
ANSWER: b

NOTES
• Somatostatin inhibits release of both glucagon and insulin from the pancreas. Somatostatin also reduces stimulated gastric acid secretion and CCK-induced gallbladder contraction.
• Somatostatin delays gastric emptying and reduces pancreatic exocrine secretion. Growth hormone secretion is inhibited.

• Somatostatinomas present with a characteristic triad of gallstones, diarrhoea and steatorrhoea. Plasma immunoreactive somatostatin levels are usually >10 times normal in cases of somatostatinoma. Arginine or tolbutamide may enhance equivocal levels.

SLEISENGER & FORDTRAN (1993) pp. 31, 1709

254. Infective diarrhoea and antimicrobial drugs
ANSWERS: c e

NOTES

• Antibiotic treatment is not generally effective in non-typhoidal Salmonella enteritis and the incidence and duration of intestinal carriage are increased following antibiotic treatment. Ampicillin or trimethoprim–sulphonamide is acceptable in cases of severe systemic infection.

• Antibiotic treatment is effective in severe diarrhoea due to *Shigella flexneri*. Ampicillin, tetracyclines or quinolones are all effective.

• *Campylobacter jejuni* is sensitive to erythromycin *in vitro* but studies fail to show a clinical benefit. Faecal excretion of *Campylobacter* is reduced by erythromycin treatment. Penicillins, cephalosporins or sulphonamides have little effect.

• *Salmonella typhi* is generally sensitive to chloramphenicol and ampicillin.

• Both ciprofloxacin and trimethoprim–sulphamethoxazole have been shown to reduce the incidence of travellers' diarrhoea.

• Diarrhoea due to *Clostridium difficile* is ameliorated by vancomycin or metronidazole.

SLEISENGER & FORDTRAN (1993) p. 1128

255. Gastrointestinal infection with leucocytes and red cells on faecal microscopy
ANSWER: b

NOTES

• Toxigenic infections cause diarrhoea without mucosal invasion and are not associated with leucocytes and red cells on faecal microscopy. The diarrhoea is characteristically watery and pain is diffuse and periumbilical.

- Toxigenic infections include:

(a) enteropathogenic *Escherichia coli* (EPEC)

(b) enterotoxigenic *E. coli* (ETEC)

(c) *Vibrio cholerae*

(d) rotavirus

(e) *Giardia lamblia*.

- Invasive colonic infections causing dysentery with leucocytes and red cells on faecal microscopy include:

(a) *Campylobacter jejuni*

(b) *Shigella*

(c) enteroinvasive *E. coli* (EIEC)

(d) enterohaemorrhagic *E. coli* (EHEC).

- Variable findings with respect to faecal leucocytes occur in:

(a) non-typhoidal salmonella

(b) *Yersinia* infections

(c) *Vibrio parahaemolyticus*

(d) *Clostridium difficile*.

- Amoebic dysentry is associated with a paucity of white cells in the stool.

SLEISENGER & FORDTRAN (1993) p. 1156

256. Hepatitis B serology
ANSWER: a

NOTES

- HBsAg is an antigen present in the outer coat of HBV. The identification of HBsAg in the serum almost always indicates active HBV infection. In the majority of patients HBsAg becomes negative within 20 weeks. HBsAg-negative HBV infection occurs in about 25% and is usually associated with clinically mild disease.

- HBsAg is usually present before icterus is clinically evident in acute HBV hepatitis.

- HBeAg is detected only in the serum of patients in whom HBsAg is also present. It is seen soon after transaminase levels peak (i.e. later than HBsAg) and is related to the presence of the core particle and HBV DNA polymerase.

- HBV DNA polymerase activity has been demonstrated only in sera which are positive for HBeAg. HBeAg in chronic carriers indicates infectivity; anti-HBe antibody indicates the opposite.

241

• Anti-HBs antibody is present in the serum of convalescent patients, vaccinated subjects and carriers.

• HBcAg is not detected in acute cases but anti-HBc antibody develops during acute infection and persists for some years in most patients. High levels of anti-HBcAg occur in chronic carriers.

• Patients with HBsAg present for more than 20 weeks are likely to remain positive for a prolonged period (chronic carriers). About 10% of chronic carriers cease to be HBeAg-positive each year that they are followed. The rate of reversion of HBsAg positivity is lower (about 2% per year).

MANDELL, BENNETT & DOLIN (1995) p. 1209

257. Q fever
ANSWERS: b e

NOTES
• *Coxiella burnetii* is the causative organism of Q fever. It differs from rickettsiae since it is more resistant to drying, heating and chemical attack and does not cross-react with *Proteus* antigen (the Weil–Felix reaction).

• Humans are the only animal in whom it causes a recognizable disease. Non-specific features predominate, including fever, malaise, myalgia and meningism. A severe headache is characteristic but rash is unusual and sparse when present. There is a dry cough but respiratory features are not usually prominent, although severe atypical pnumonia is recognized.

• Complications include endocarditis (especially aortic valve) and granulomatous hepatitis.

• Infection is common in domestic animals (especially cattle, sheep and goats but including cats, dogs and a wide variety of other animals). The organism is excreted in milk and in placentas.

• Most transmission appears to result from inhalation of organisms in dust (farm workers and abattoir workers have a particular risk). Drinking of raw contaminated milk is a documented source of infection.

• Person-to-person infection is documented (but rare). Laboratory staff are at risk if culturing the organism.

• Complement fixation tests are most commonly used in diagnosis.

• Tetracycline is the treatment of choice. Rifampicin and quinolones are possible alternatives or additions. Erythromycin appears ineffective.

MANDELL, BENNETT & DOLIN (1995) p. 1473

258. Protein C deficiency
ANSWER: all incorrect

NOTES
• Inheritance is autosomal dominant. Affected patients have approximately 50% of normal protein C concentrations.
• Most patients are asymptomatic until the second or third decade, from which time recurrent venous thromboses and pulmonary embolism occur.
• Protein C is a vitamin K-dependent protease which complements antithrombin III action by inhibiting factor Va and VIIIa activity and increasing fibrin degredation.
• Routine coagulation tests are normal. Protein C may be assayed using a chromogenic assay.
• Warfarin is required on a long-term basis. Following initiation of therapy, antithrombin III levels may be further decreased (since protein C is vitamin K-dependent): this may be associated with a transient increase in thrombosis. Consequently initiation of warfarin should be covered by heparin.
• Protein C levels increase during pregnancy. Androgens significantly raise protein levels and may be effective therapeutically.

LEE *et al.* (1993) p. 1522

259. Antithrombin III
ANSWERS: a d e

NOTES
• Antithrombin III deficiency is inherited as an autosomal dominant.
• Antithrombin III is an α-globulin which is a major inhibitor of the coagulation cascade, especially of thrombin. Binding of antithrombin III is enhanced 1000 times by complexing with heparin.
• Recurrent thrombosis and thromboembolism occur from the second or third decade in patients with antithrombin III deficiency, but are rare before puberty. Arterial thrombi are rare.

- Pregnancy and oral contraceptives are very significant risk factors for women with antithrombin III deficiency.
- Antithrombin III is present in fresh frozen plasma and levels can be increased by fresh frozen plasma infusion.
- Oral anticoagulant treatment is associated with increased anti-thrombin III levels while heparin is associated with decreased levels.
- Thromboses complicating antithrombin III deficiency generally respond poorly to heparin. Androgens increase antithrombin III levels.

LEE *et al.* (1993) p. 1520

260. *Entamoeba histolytica*
ANSWER: e

NOTES
- *Entamoeba histolytica* cysts are excreted in the faeces of infected persons and can survive for some weeks in a favourable environment. Ingestion of cysts results in excystation in the small bowel and trophozoite infection in the colon.
- Encystment occurs in the colon while excreted trophozoites degenerate very rapidly outside the body.
- Amoebae invade the colonic mucosa and may result in hepatic abscesses by way of the portal vein. Haem-positive stools are the rule. Faecal leucocytes are present but are less numerous than is the case in bacillary dysentry.
- Fulminant colitis is an unusual presentation but colonic perforations are associated with this form of disease. More commonly, there is a presentation with chronic diarrhoea and abdominal pain.
- Most patients who develop liver abscess present within 6 months of leaving an endemic area. Amoebae are present on microscopy in the stools of <40% of cases. There is a leucocytosis but no eosinophilia.

MANDELL, BENNETT & DOLIN (1995) p. 2395

Index

proximal tubule of nephron, **52**, (220–221)
pruritus, **22–23**, (131)
pseudohypoparathyroidism type I, **12**, (98)
psittacosis (ornithosis), **10**, (92)
psoriasis, **20**, (122)
  arthropathy, **24**, (134)
ptosis, **2**, (64)
pulmonary embolism, **49**, (213–214)
pyloric stenosis, results of vomiting, **36**, (173)
pyogenic meningitis, **27–28**, (146–147)

Q fever, **59**, (242–243)

rabies, **33**, (164)
reflexes, extensor plantar with absent knee jerks, **21**, (127–128)
Reiter's syndrome, **29–30**, (153)
renal fluid handling, **28**, (147–148)
rheumatic fever, **23**, (133)
rubella, **9–10**, (90)

Salmenella typhi, **2**, (63–64)
sarcoidosis, **56–57**, (235–236)
Schistosoma haematobium, **39**, (181–182)
scleroderma, **16–17**, (112–113)
secretin, **39**, (183)
secretin test, **39**, (182)
segmental demyelination, **57**, (236–237)
sexual precocity, **52**, (222–223)
short stature, **24**, (135)
sickle-cell disease
  anaemia (homozygote), **8**, (83–84)
  trait (heterozygote), **11**, (94–95)
sideroblastic anaemia, **46–47**, (206–207)
Sjögren's syndrome, **40–41**, (187)
skin disorders
  malignant disease, **20**, (123–124)
  oral lesions, **52**, (221)
somatostatin, **58**, (239–240)

spinal cord
  anatomy, **46**, (204)
  damage, Brown-Séquard syndrome, **9**, (88–89)
splenectomy, **36**, (174–175)
steatorrhoea, **45**, (201)
subacute infective endocarditis, **4–5**, (72–73)
syphilis
  Argyll Robertson pupils, **46**, (203–204)
  serology, **54–55**, (229–230)
  tabes dorsalis, **6**, (77)
syringomyelia, **10**, (92–93)
systemic lupus erythematosus (SLE), **2**, **11**, (64–65), (96)
systemic sclerosis (scleroderma), **16–17**, (112–113)

tabes dorsalis, **6**, (77)
tamoxifen, **31–32**, (159)
tardive dyskinesia, **43**, (194–195)
target cells, **37**, (177)
Tay–Sachs disease, **24**, (136)
tetralogy of Fallot, **19**, (120)
thiamine deficiency (beriberi), **6**, (78–79)
thrombolytic therapy, **16**, (112)
torsade de pointes, **57–58**, (239)
toxic shock syndrome (TSS), **36–37**, (175)
Toxoplasma gondii, **54**, (227–228)
trisomy 21 (Down's syndrome), **51**, (219)

ulcerative colitis, **41**, (189–190)
ulnar nerve, **42–43**, (192–193)
uricosuric drugs, **20–21**, (125)
urinary sediment, **18**, (118)
urine reducing substances, **23**, (132–133)

varicella, **32–33**, (162)
variegate porphyria, **18**, (118)
vascular 'spider' telangiectasia, **31**, (157)
visual pathway, **37–38**, (178)

249